Phantom Pain

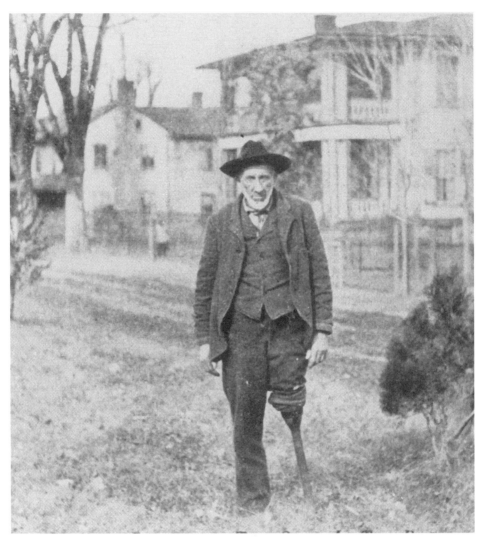

Samuel Eller of Rowan County, a private in Company H, Twenty-third North Carolina Troops, was shot three times in the leg on July 1, 1863, at Gettysburg. The severity of his wounds required the removal of the damaged limb. The state provided Eller with a Jewett artificial leg on July 3, 1866. In this 1909 photograph, he is wearing another type of prosthesis, the Jewett leg, no doubt, having worn out long before. Eller's image appeared on the cover of the July 1998 *North Carolina Historical Review*. This book serves as an expansion of Ansley Herring Wegner's article therein, titled "Phantom Pain: Civil War Amputation and North Carolina's Maimed Veterans." Image courtesy of State Archives, North Carolina Office of Archives and History. Raleigh.

Phantom Pain

North Carolina's Artificial-Limbs
Program for Confederate Veterans

Including an Index to Records
in the North Carolina State Archives
Related to Artificial Limbs for Confederate Veterans

Ansley Herring Wegner

Office of Archives and History
North Carolina Department of Cultural Resources
Raleigh
2004

COVER: Confederate veterans from Catawba County from a photograph taken in the early twentieth century. They are, from left to right, George W. Rabb, J. U. Long, Henry J. Reitzel, and J. M. Arndt. Rabb, Reitzel, and Arndt were members of Company A, Twelfth North Carolina Troops. Long served in Company F, Thirty-second North Carolina Troops. Image courtesy of the Catawba County Museum of History Archive. Cover design by Darryl Ketcham.

Contents

Illustrations

Foreword

Wounds to the extremities ranked among the most common in the American Civil War, accounting for 71 percent of all injuries to Union soldiers. Large-caliber Civil War muskets and rifles fired conoidal minié balls at a low velocity. On impact these tended to flatten, shattering bones and lodging in the target's body rather than passing through it. Infection soon followed. Civil War surgeons, frequently hurried, overworked, and under trained, often performed surgery far from well-appointed hospitals. Under such circumstances, they commonly resorted to amputations to check gangrene, osteomyelitis, or septicemia in lesions that resulted from wounds.

As a result, amputations constituted roughly 75 percent of all operations performed during the Civil War. Of the 29,980 amputations performed on Union soldiers, 21,753 men survived. The 26 percent mortality rate for Federal amputees was 2 percent lower than that of patients treated by what were then considered to be more conservative remedies.

Ansley Herring Wegner's painstaking and pioneering research fills a void in the medical and social history of North Carolina's Confederate amputees and maimed veterans. Surveying amputation's place in Victorian medical science, and the problems disabled veterans confronted as they reentered civilian life, she argues that "North Carolina was unwavering in her attempt to aid and support the maimed Confederate veterans."

Though North Carolina, like other former Confederate states, experienced severe economic difficulties during Reconstruction, in early 1866 the state nevertheless legislated funds to provide amputees "necessary [artificial] limbs, and thus to restore them, as far as practicable, to the comfortable use of their persons, to the enjoyment of life and to the ability to earn a subsistence." During the war and its aftermath inventors patented several types of artificial limbs.

After examining North Carolina's program to supply and fit its Confederate amputees with artificial arms and legs, Wegner explains the response of recipients to their new limbs. Some adjusted to the prostheses, she states, while others suffered from residual ailments associated with stumps that never healed properly. Many reported phantom pain from the amputated region. Wegner also compares North Carolina's artificial-limbs program with that of other former Confederate states. She concludes that North Carolina was among the most progressive and forthcoming of the southern states in supporting its disabled and maimed former Confederate soldiers.

In January 1866, a Raleigh newspaper endorsed enthusiastically state-funded artificial limbs for North Carolina's former Confederate soldiers. "The State owes them, at least, this small token of her appreciation . . . prompted by humane and honorable motives." Wegner's compact and thoughtful study reminds us of the debt North Carolinians owed their veterans as they reflected on the horrors and sacrifices of war and the vicissitudes of peace.

John David Smith
Charles H. Stone Distinguished Professor of American History
University of North Carolina at Charlotte

Acknowledgments

In a project of this scope and duration, debts of gratitude accumulate. I began arranging the papers of the Artificial Limbs Department while I was a reference archivist in the North Carolina State Archives. As my work progressed, I grew curious about the artificial-limbs program. What sort of limbs were available? Why, at a time of economic hardship, was North Carolina willing to spend so much money on wooden legs? My supervisor at the time, C. Edward Morris, permitted me to pursue the extensive work that I envisioned. Druscie Simpson found a computer for me when my note-card index of amputees proved unwieldy. Dr. John David Smith shared with me his research on the rehabilitation of amputees. Once I moved to my present position as a historian in the Research Branch, my supervisor, Michael Hill, generously allowed me to continue working on the manuscript and provided help by reading drafts and making suggestions. Lang Baradell, my editor, offered invaluable assistance in improving the text. His meticulous review of the table of veterans was extraordinary. Susan Trimble deserves credit for her conscientious typesetting. The lengthy table was an exceedingly difficult undertaking. Lisa Bailey contributed her masterful skills as a proofreader. Alan Westmoreland has been a tremendous asset to this project, not only for his photography, but for driving to Red Springs to pick up the Jewett leg from Duncan Hanna. Len Hambleton, conservator at the North Carolina Museum of History, graciously repaired and performed conservation work on the Hanna leg to prepare it for photographs for the book and to facilitate an examination of the interior of the leg. Ultimately, it was Duncan Hanna who contributed something tangible to my years of research when he agreed to lend me his grandfather's artificial leg to study and photograph. Access to that leg, in addition to being the ideal culmination to my research, has provided a substantive connection with the hardships endured by the amputees.

Phantom Pain

The Industrial Revolution in America had a profound and complex impact on the Civil War. Telegraphs, steamships, and railroads, by heightening communication and mobility, increased enlistment and improved support services for troops. Telegraphs expedited communication between commanders and accelerated the deployment of soldiers. Railroads and steamships efficiently moved men and supplies, enabling the amassing of larger armies and lengthening the time troops could remain in the field.

Technological advancements prior to and during the Civil War also furnished soldiers with firearms that were more destructive than any previously used by Americans. A new process in the manufacture of weapons called rifling—the placement of grooves inside the barrel—caused projectiles to follow a truer trajectory, thus increasing accuracy at greater distances. The standard-issue bullet during the Civil War was the soft-lead, expansive minié ball. Developed by members of the French army and introduced in 1849, the minié ball would flatten upon impact and cause gaping wounds. While most Civil War soldiers used muzzle-loaders, some troops were issued breech-loading rifles. These new weapons shortened loading time and increased the number of bullets a soldier could fire in battle. These and other innovations produced an unprecedented increase in the frequency and severity of injuries.

The failure of officers to change military tactics, despite the modifications in armaments, also contributed to the growth of casualty rates. Many Civil War generals had learned their trade during the Mexican War, when weapons were still smooth-bore and largely inaccurate at a range exceeding a hundred yards. This inaccuracy, combined with the time-consuming process of loading a muzzle-loader, meant that charging troops usually had to endure only one volley of accurate fire before reaching the enemy. Rifling increased the distance at which a weapon could be fired accurately by three to four times. As a result, Civil War soldiers charging across open fields were

TABLE 1

Consolidated Table of Amputations, from June 1, 1862, to February 1, 1864, collated from Reports in the Surgeon-General's Office.

	Primary				Secondary			
	Cases	Cures	Deaths	Percent	Cases	Cures	Deaths	Percent
Thigh	345	213	132	38	162	43	119	73
Leg	314	219	95	30	150	76	74	49
Arm	294	252	42	14	140	87	53	37
Forearm	69	61	8	12	45	35	10	22
Shoulder-joint	79	54	25	31	28	8	20	71
Elbow-joint	4	3	1	25	3	2	1	-
Wrist-joint	7	5	2	28	-	-	-	-
Hip-joint	3	1	2	66	-	-	-	-
Knee-joint	5	2	3	60	6	-	6	100
Ankle-joint	6	4	2	33	4	4	-	-
Tarsal-joint	16	13	3	19	8	7	1	12
Total	1149*	827	315	27	546	262	284	51

SOURCE: John Julian Chisolm, *A Manual of Military Surgery*, 3d. ed. (1864; reprint, Dayton, Ohio: Morningside Press, 1992), 361.

* The actual number of cases totaled 1142 and not 1149.

subjected to accurate fire sooner and for longer periods of time.[1] Despite the resulting increase in casualties, generals were slow to abandon their methods and continued to send infantry head-on against heavily defended positions.

Doctors had neither the experience nor technology to adequately repair the shattered limbs and mangled bodies that were more quickly amassed by the larger armies and more potent weaponry. Moreover, because Civil War surgeons had to care for so many wounded, they often did not have the time to perform tedious reconstructive operations. Thus, amputations and resectioning of joints—that is, the removal of bone—became standard practice. While amputations had been performed for centuries, sterilization and post-surgical infections were still not yet understood. Despite the imprecise procedures and frenzied, unsanitary conditions, the survival rate for amputees was surprisingly high. [See Table 1] This left large numbers of maimed veterans trying to make their way in the economically devastated postbellum South.

1. Gerald F. Linderman, *Embattled Courage: The Experience of Combat in the Civil War* (New York: Free Press, 1987), 135.

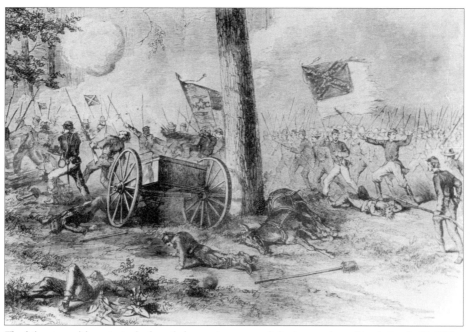

The failure to modify tactics in the face of advances in weaponry led to increased casualties during the Civil War. Newly developed rifled weapons made frontal assaults, common in earlier wars, more costly. This image of the Battle of Bentonville appears in Paul F. Mottelay and T. Campbell-Copeland, eds. , *The Soldier in Our Civil War: A Pictorial History of the Conflict, 1861-1865*, v. 2 (New York: Stanley Bradley, 1890), 362. In that version, however, the Confederate and North Carolina banners are United States flags. Image courtesy of State Archives.

Confederate amputees obviously found their lives irrevocably altered. The hero's welcome faded as southerners memorialized their dead and contended with the war's emotional and economic consequences. Phantom pain, the ghostly sensation of pain from a missing limb, vexed the maimed soldiers as the ghosts of the dead haunted the South. Perhaps to capitalize on southern loyalties and sympathies, Confederate amputees initially made no effort to hide their wounds. They pinned up their shirt sleeves and pants legs proudly and were heard to make statements such as "at least I lived" or "it was a small price to pay for the cause."

North Carolina quickly became a leader among southern states in providing artificial limbs or, for those who could not use prostheses, monetary commutations to its maimed Confederate veterans. The policies for the program, the first of its kind among the former Confederate states, changed and grew with the public's support. But despite postwar economic hardships, North Carolina unwaveringly provided assistance. The result constituted a noble effort by North Carolina's government to assist the maimed survivors of the "lost cause" to once again become productive members of their communities. In reality, however, providing limbs and commutations proved to be more of a psychological than economic benefit to the veterans. Even in that regard, the state's largesse could not erase the bitterness among some veterans over the price that they had already paid for that piece of cork or willow sculpted into the shape of their missing appendage.

A Brief History of American Medicine

To put North Carolina's artificial-limbs program in context, the evolution of American medicine and prosthetics should be considered. During the nation's early years, physicians learned their trade primarily through apprenticeships. The student paid a fee to live and work with a doctor for two to five years.[2] A few medical schools existed, but the general public distrusted them because they were known to procure bodies for dissection by robbing graves. As the country's population increased, however, the number of medical schools multiplied to meet the growing demand for medical care. By 1810, some medical schools, usually those unaffiliated with a college, no longer considered medical training or laboratory work necessary for a degree. All that was needed to found these proprietary schools was a charter, lecturers, and a building in which to hold classes. There were few entrance requirements, and degrees were easily obtained.[3] The quality of the education depended on the instructors who, for the most part, were products of apprenticeships and lacked formal medical training themselves.

Also in the early nineteenth century, state medical societies began to establish examination boards to license physicians. Because board members were paid only when a license was granted, the system was rife with corruption. The boards in some states accepted medical degrees, even those from the inferior proprietary schools, as grounds for automatic licensing. Furthermore, in the wave of Jacksonian egalitarianism in the 1820s and early 1830s, many Americans believed that they, and not a board, should decide who could be their doctor.[4] This and the growing need for medical practitioners led to the lifting of most restrictions and licensing measures. Thus, by the beginning of the Civil War, no medical licensing system existed in America.

Prior to the war, the surgical experience of most American doctors consisted of minor procedures, such as extracting teeth and lancing boils, with sporadic trauma cases.[5] French surgeons by this time, however, having learned that many ailments were accompanied by lesions on organs, had begun to surgically remove diseased organs. Some American doctors, especially those on the frontier, had experimented with this treatment, but because methods were crude and patients fearful, surgery was not the preferred treatment.[6]

Surgery became more practical in the 1840s with the discovery of safe, reliable anesthetics. Ether, previously known only as a solvent, was first used during an

2. John Duffy, *The Healers: A History of American Medicine* (Urbana: University of Illinois Press, 1979), 166.

3. Duffy, *Healers*, 170-172.

4. Duffy, *Healers*, 176-177.

5. Duffy, *Healers*, 220.

6. H. H. Cunningham, *Doctors in Gray* (1958; reprint, Baton Rouge: Louisiana State University Press, 1993), 18-19.

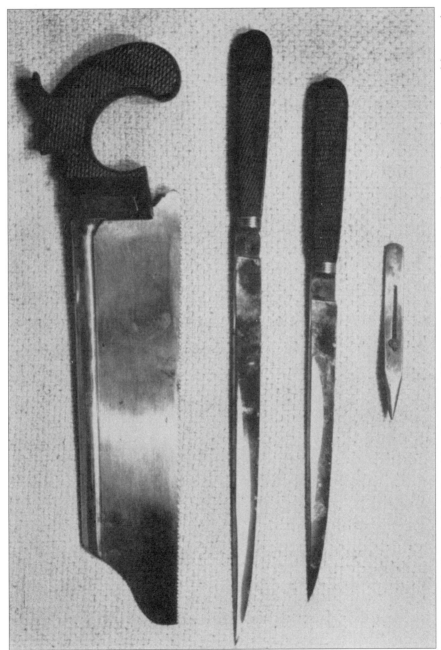

Dr. Edmund Burke Haywood of Raleigh used these instruments while a surgeon in the Confederate army. The two knives in the center and the saw at the top were used to amputate limbs. Image from H. H. Cunningham, "Edmund Burke Haywood and Raleigh's Confederate Hospitals," *North Carolina Historical Review* 35 (April 1958): facing 165.

operation by Crawford Williamson Long of Georgia in 1842. William Thomas Green Morton of Massachusetts also did extensive research on ether as an anesthetic during the same period. On October 16, 1846, Morton stimulated interest in ether as an anesthetic by conducting a public demonstration at Massachusetts General Hospital. Inspired by the successful use of ether in America, James Simpson of Edinburgh, Scotland, conducted experiments with other forms of anesthesia. In 1847, he introduced chloroform as an anesthetic.

Anesthesia enabled doctors to perform longer and more complex operations. These prolonged surgeries, however, coupled with unsanitary conditions, led to increased incidences of gangrene and other surgical infections. Benjamin Winslow Dudley, a professor of medicine at Kentucky's Transylvania University Medical School from 1817 to 1850, learned that using boiled water to thoroughly cleanse the "surgical field" before and after surgery decreased post-surgical infections. Although Dudley taught his students to follow this procedure, it was not standard practice by the time of the Civil War. Joseph Lister would not publish his now famous works on antiseptics until 1867, too late for Civil War surgeons and patients.[7] Thus, with little surgical experience or medical knowledge, young doctors, many unlicensed, enlisted in the medical corps to be faced with the extensive surgical needs of the Confederate wounded.

A Brief History of Amputation and Artificial Limbs

The oldest testimony to human amputation of extremities is a thirty-six-thousand-year-old imprint of a hand, apparently with two fingers amputated, on a cave wall in Spain. Prehistoric bones have been discovered that show evidence of amputation, and prehistoric tools of stone and bone resembling animals' jaws have been demonstrated to be capable of removing a limb in six minutes. Early amputations were primarily conducted as religious rites or punishment.[8] The best example of the latter can be found in the practices of pre-Incan Indians in what is now Peru. Around 1500 B.C.E., this society lived under laws forbidding lying, stealing, and laziness. The punishment for the first of these transgressions was the removal of lips and nose; the second, the amputation of a hand; and the third, amputation of a foot.[9]

All documented early amputations were conducted by quickly removing the limb in a sawing motion to prevent the patient from dying of shock. Surprisingly, the

7. Julian E. Kuz and Bradley P. Bengston, *Orthopaedic Injuries of the Civil War* (Kennesaw, Ga.: Kennesaw Mountain Press, 1996), 9.

8. Lawrence W. Friedman, *The Psychological Rehabilitation of the Amputee* (Springfield, Ill.: Charles C. Thomas, 1978), 3-5.

9. Friedman, *Psychological Rehabilitation*, 6-7.

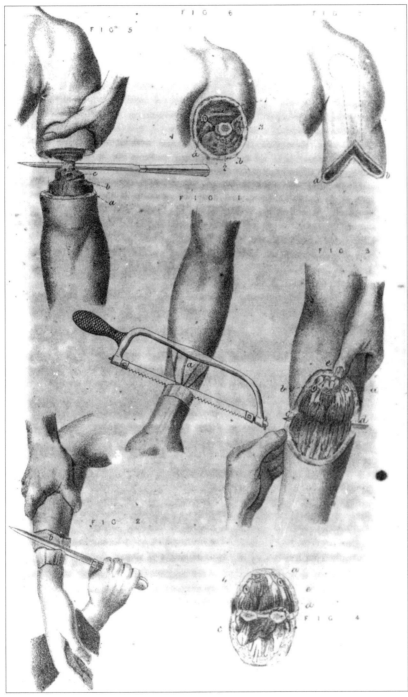

Before the Civil War, most doctors performed only minor surgical procedures. The carnage of the battlefield, however, forced them to learn quickly how to operate in the worst of conditions on wounds unlike any encountered in peacetime. This is a page from one of their instruction books, A *Manual of Military Surgery*, showing methods of amputation. Image courtesy of State Archives.

resulting blood loss rarely caused death.[10] Such amputations were often left to heal by granulation, the body's natural healing process by which new capillaries and thick tissue form over the wound, much like a scab, to protect the wound. This method, in fact, was prevalent during the Civil War, since surgeons rarely had time to tie off the interrupted blood vessels.

Those who survived amputation and the resulting infections sought artificial limbs for functional and ornamental reasons. Because of the need for mobility, crutches and, subsequently, artificial legs appear to have developed more than one thousand years before artificial arms. More than three thousand years ago, simple stick crutches began to evolve into peg-type prostheses, which were either held and guided by a cane-like extension to the hand or strapped to the stump with leather braces. The first true advances in prosthetic technology occurred during the Middle Ages. Armorers developed iron legs, arms, and hands for knights to use in battle. These were functional, in that they helped the amputee to fight, as well as cosmetic, in hiding evidence of limb loss, which would have implied failure in a previous battle.[11]

In 1861, on the eve of the Civil War, a committee of surgeons published a report on the current technology in artificial legs. The report's author, Dr. James M. Minor, declared, "In walking, [power, speed, and adaptation] are brought into rapid, varied, and beautifully harmonious action, such as can only be imperfectly imitated by the most ingenious mechanism of man's contrivance."[12] The primary leg designs included in the report were the Anglesea, Bly, Palmer, and Jewett legs. The committee concluded that the Anglesea and Bly products were superior to the others. Jewett's Patent Leg was praised, however, for its "mechanical perfection and simplicity of arrangement" and for the ease with which it could be repaired.[13]

An 1864 article in the *Confederate States Medical and Surgical Journal* stated that the Jewett leg, while cosmetically appealing, was too heavy and generally inferior to the Palmer and Bly legs, both of which employed exceptional ankle joints.[14] The article went on to encourage locksmiths, gunsmiths, toolmakers, and others who were mechanically inclined to develop artificial limbs to fill the seemingly endless demand. It should be noted that the Palmer, Bly, and Jewett legs were manufactured in the North, while the Anglesea leg was made in England. The Confederacy thus desperately needed to foster production of artificial limbs, just as it did with many other industrial products.

---

10. Roberto H. Barja and Richard A. Sherman, *What to Expect When You Lose A Limb* (Washington, D.C.: U.S. Government Printing Office, 1986), 5.

11. Friedman, *Psychological Rehabilitation*, 10.

12. James M. Minor, "Report on Artificial Limbs," *Bulletin of the New York Academy of Medicine* 1 (1861): 165.

13. Minor, "Report on Artificial Limbs," 172, 173.

14. "Artificial Limbs and How to Make Them," *Confederate States Medical and Surgical Journal* 1 (April 1864): 59.

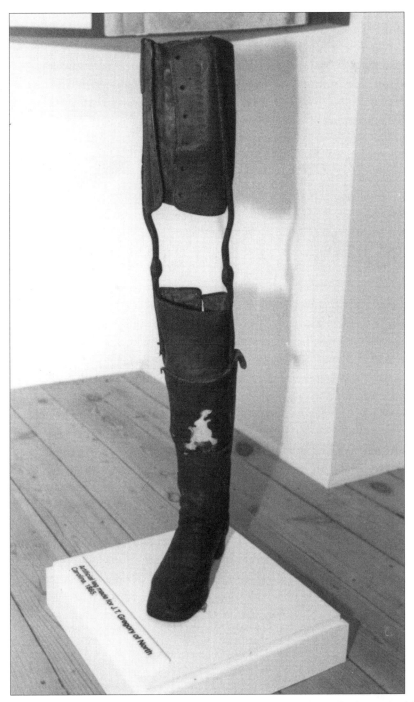

John T. Gregory of Sampson County, a veteran of the Third Arkansas, obtained this artificial leg in Charlottesville, Virginia, in 1865, before North Carolina provided limbs to veterans. Satisfied with it, and having no need for a second artificial leg, Gregory requested and received the seventy-dollar commutation from North Carolina in 1866. The leg is on display at Bennet Place State Historic Site near Durham, North Carolina. Photograph by Alan Westmoreland. Image courtesy of State Archives.

From 1846 to 1860, thirty-four patents for new or improved prosthetic devices and invalid chairs, or wheelchairs, were registered. From 1861 to 1873, the number grew to 133 patents, a 290 percent increase. Eighty-eight of these patents were for artificial legs, nineteen for crutches, eight for invalid chairs, and eighteen for arms and hands.[15] During the mid-nineteenth century, just as throughout human history, the amputee's need for mobility was the driving force in the technical modifications of artificial limbs.

Combat Surgery and Battle Wounds

> Modern warfare, in introducing arms of precision, of immensely
> increased range, and perfected instruments of destruction of heavy
> calibre, has created a new era in military surgery.[16]
>
> –J. Julian Chisolm
> A Manual of Military Surgery (1864)

Statistics show that 94 percent of battle wounds in the Civil War were from bullets and that the most widely used bullet was the newly developed minié ball—a conical-shaped projectile made from soft lead. Because of the low velocity generated by the muskets and the tendency of the minié ball to flatten upon impact, the resulting wounds were often large and ragged.[17] J. Julian Chisolm, a Charleston, South Carolina, physician and professor of surgery at the Medical College of South Carolina, wrote A Manual of Military Surgery. In it he stated that should minié balls "impinge upon the bone, the splitting and crushing is so extensive as to necessitate more frequently amputations and resections."[18]

As it was commonly recognized that a wounded soldier was a greater handicap to his army than a dead one, troops were frequently instructed to shoot to wound, not to kill.[19] Once wounded, soldiers were at the mercy of medical staff members whose methods had not kept pace with the destructive technological advances in weaponry. When the wounded soldier was retrieved from the field by the ambulance corps, he generally received first aid in the form of whiskey or, when available, opium.[20] Because wound dressings would be removed at the field hospital, bandages were applied on the battlefield only in cases of severe bleeding in order to conserve materials. Tourniquets

15. Laurann Figg and Jane Farrell-Beck, "Amputation in the Civil War: Physical and Social Dimensions" (unpublished manuscript, Vesterheim Museum, Decorah, Iowa, 1993), 7.

16. J. Julian Chisolm, A Manual of Military Surgery, 3d ed. (1864; reprint, Dayton: Morningside Press, 1992), 119.

17. Duffy, Healers, 220.

18. Chisolm, Manual of Military Surgery, 119.

19. Cunningham, Doctors in Gray, 219.

20. Duffy, Healers, 221.

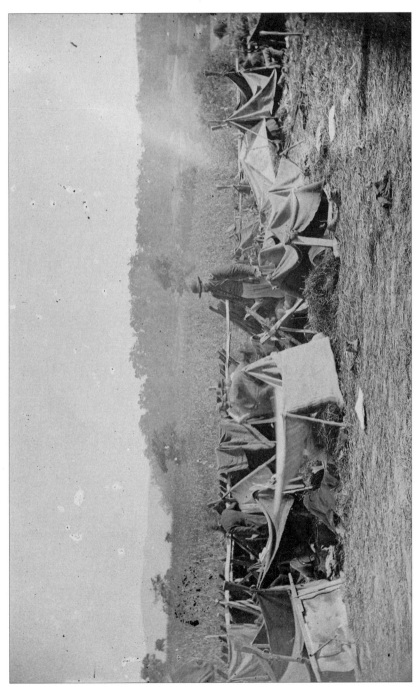

Doctors tended patients, often from both armies, under abysmal conditions in the field. In this primitive makeshift hospital, a Union doctor treats Confederates wounded at the Battle of Antietam. Alexander Gardner, "Keedysville, Md., vicinity, Confederate wounded at Smith's Barn, with Dr. Anson Hurd, 14th Indiana Volunteers in attendance," September 1862, Civil War Photographs, 1861-1865, Library of Congress (http://memory.loc.gov/cgi-bin/query/D?cwar:8:./temp/~ammem_MhzL::), January 14, 2004.

were rarely used because of the potential for damage to the limb. If the correct pressure point could be located, an attendant would plug the wound with his finger.[21]

Once the wounded soldier was placed in the field infirmary, a surgeon thoroughly examined the wound. When possible the doctor pinned a note to the soldier's clothes describing his conclusions in order to prevent further examinations that could harm the patient. As Chisolm explained, "After-examinations heighten irritation and inflammation in the wound, and, as they permit air (which ought to be rigorously excluded) to pass through to the bottom of the wound, this promotes the decomposition of extravasated fluids and exudations, [and] induces suppuration and sloughing."[22]

The examination would begin with the soldier's clothing. By careful observation the doctor could identify a bullet's entry point, possibly an exit point, and whether or not any torn clothing might be lodged in the wound. The next step was to locate the bullet and any other foreign objects. "As the patient is now faint from loss of blood and from nervous depression," Chisolm explained, "the wound not yet being painful or swollen, the surgeon, using his finger—which is the only admissible probe on such occasions that the military surgeon of experience recognizes—examines with it, if possible, the entire extent of the wound, searching for foreign bodies."[23]

With this, the best examination possible, completed, the wound was dressed, preferably with cotton or lint. The patient was then ready for what was frequently a traumatic journey to the nearest hospital. The wounded were often moved in wagons over rough roads or in filthy railroad cars that had been used to transport livestock.[24] Kate Cumming, a volunteer Confederate nurse, in describing the transporting of wounded by wagon concluded, "All this was very trying to the wounded, and the wonder to me is how they could live after such a ride, for it was really harrowing."[25]

Once at the hospital, particularly after a difficult journey, the wounded soldier would be treated for shock. Before any surgery, the doctor would warm the patient's body and strengthen his pulse by wrapping him in blankets or warm clothes and administering wine, brandy, or whiskey to restore "nervous energy."[26] If surgery was to be performed, whether amputation, as was most common, or a resection or other repair, the patient was anesthetized with ether or chloroform. The latter was preferred because of the ease with which it could be administered.[27] Chisolm considered

---

21. Chisolm, *Manual of Military Surgery*, 171.

22. Chisolm, *Manual of Military Surgery*, 149.

23. Chisolm, *Manual of Military Surgery*, 172.

24. Bell I. Wiley, *The Life of Johnny Reb* (Baton Rouge: Louisiana State University, 1994), 263-264.

25. Kate Cumming, *Kate: The Journal of a Confederate Nurse*, ed. Richard Barksdale Harwell (Baton Rouge: Louisiana State University Press, 1959), 156.

26. Chisolm, *Manual of Military Surgery*, 151.

27. Duffy, *Healers*, 221.

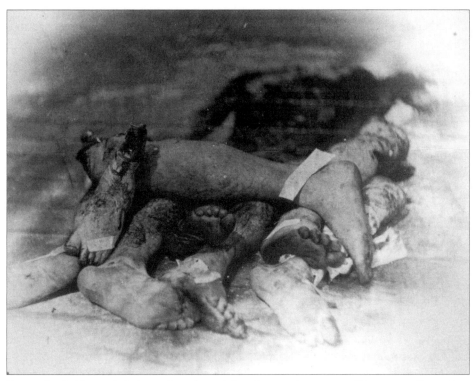

Doctors, faced with overwhelming numbers of wounded, used amputation as an expeditious means of increasing a critically wounded soldier's chances for survival. Consequently, piles of severed limbs were a common sight at field hospitals. Image courtesy of National Museum of Health and Medicine, Armed Forces Institute of Pathology, Washington, D.C., Photograph CP 1043.

chloroform a product of the "humanizing tendencies of the age" that had "banished that dread of being cut."[28] While this might be an exaggeration, chloroform was considered to be indispensable in military surgical practice during the Civil War.

The surgeon had to decide quickly if amputation was necessary. Occasionally, field surgeons, if they believed that amputation was inevitable, would amputate the damaged limb in the field themselves. Some unscrupulous surgeons conducted amputations in order to gain surgical experience rather than to help the wounded.[29] Chisolm asserted that early in the war ambitious young surgeons would amputate even for the slightest flesh wounds. He noted that "the limbs of soldiers were in as much danger from the ardor of young surgeons as from the missiles of the enemy."[30] In an 1866 letter to Gov. Jonathan Worth requesting aid for a disabled veteran, Doctors

28. Chisolm, *Manual of Military Surgery*, 427, 152.

29. G. M. B. Maughs, "Thoughts on Surgery, Operative and Conservative, suggested by a visit to the Battle-field and Hospitals of the Army of Tennessee," *Confederate States Medical and Surgical Journal* 1 (September 1864): 1.

30. Chisolm, *Manual of Military Surgery*, 409.

M. L. Brown and J. M. Carson described a botched amputation. They reported that "the amputation [was] so unsuccessfully performed, and the bone protruding to such an extent that he can not bear any pressure of consequence upon it."[31]

As the war progressed, guidelines were established to determine when amputation was appropriate. These guidelines left much room for interpretation, however. For example, primary amputation, a procedure performed after shock but within twenty-four hours of the injury, was suggested in cases in which "the soft parts are much lacerated" or when the wound was so severe as to require "very tedious cures."[32] Primary amputations had a dramatically higher rate of patient survival than secondary amputations, which were generally performed within a few days of the injury. [See Table 1] Secondary amputations were to be conducted if bleeding could not be stopped or if a serious infection had developed. The lower survival rate was caused in part by blood loss but more frequently by systemic infections, which, of course, could not be stopped by the removal of an infected limb.[33]

As bad as amputations were, resectioning—the removal of bone near and possibly including the joint—could be equally disabling. A. P. Carver of Fayetteville described his experience in a letter to the governor: "I was wounded at Drewrey's Bluff My Left Arm crushed, so that I has to undergo 'resection' and have three inches of the Bone cut out Just below the shoulder Joint. Leaving the Arm hanging useless by my side, with no connection to the body except by the skin and muscles. . . . It hangs perfectly limber and can be twitched round like a piece of rope."[34] Carver went on to state that because of his good arm's overuse he injured a "tendum" and was essentially unable to work.

Chisolm recommended that after surgery patients be provided with peace and quiet while regaining strength. Toward this end, surgeons often prescribed opiates, such as morphine. Chisolm, in fact, called opium "the greatest boon to the military surgeon."[35] Kate Cumming, however, was less enthusiastic about the use of morphine. "I have been through the ward to see if the men are in need of anything," she wrote, "but all are sound asleep under the influence of morphine. Much of that is administered; more than for their good, and must injure them. I expressed this opinion to one of the doctors; he smiled, and said that it was not as bad as to let them suffer."[36] Indeed, morphine does seem preferable to the inducement of bleeding, vomiting, and purging

31. M. L. Brown and J. M. Carson to Jonathan Worth, December 20, 1866, Jonathan Worth, Governors Papers, State Archives, Office of Archives and History, Raleigh.

32. Chisolm, *Manual of Military Surgery*, 410.

33. Chisolm, *Manual of Military Surgery*, 413, 416.

34. A. P. Carver to Jonathan Worth, July 3, 1867, Jonathan Worth, Governors Papers, State Archives.

35. Chisolm, *Manual of Military Surgery*, 221.

36. Cumming, *Journal of a Confederate Nurse*, 33.

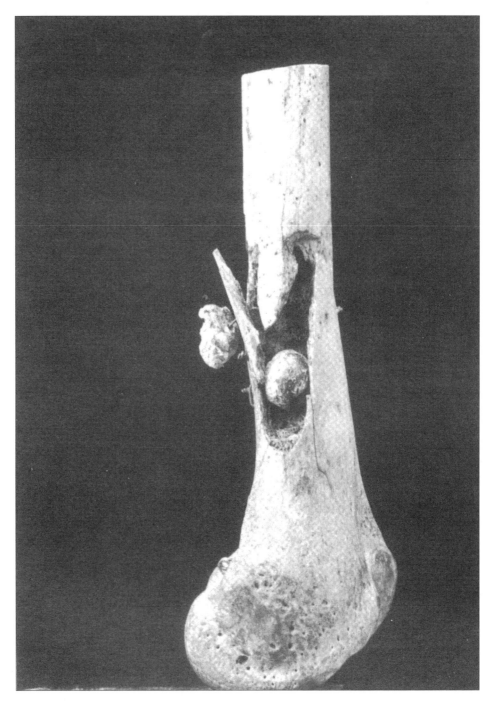

A ball fired into the thigh of a Union soldier during the Battle of Chancellorsville is still lodged in this amputated section of his left femur. The patient died of blood poisoning soon after the operation. Image courtesy of National Museum of Health and Medicine, Armed Forces Institute of Pathology, Photograph SP 163.

of the bowels, which was the standard treatment to reduce inflammation and aid recovery in military hospitals prior to the war.[37]

Because of unsanitary operating conditions and the types of surgical methods used, virtually all wounds became infected. White, creamy, "laudable" pus was expected and thought desirable because it was believed to be the body's way of expelling impurities and thus an important part of healing.[38] To stimulate the formation of pus, warm, wet dressings were often applied to wounds.[39] Since the dressings were to remain moist, they were frequently reused and rarely cleaned, which led to further spread of infection.[40]

By the time Chisolm revised his manual in 1864, he had deduced that cold water irrigation of bandages was more effective than warm water dressings.[41] A committee appointed by the Association of Army and Navy Surgeons for the Confederacy reached the same conclusion.[42] To irrigate a bandage, a water container was placed over the patient's bed with a string or strip of cloth running to the bandage as a conduit for the water. The cold water refrigerated the wound and thereby stopped the bleeding.[43] This type of dressing was generally used for about ten days but could be relied upon for up to three weeks. Once the irrigation bandage was discontinued, a local dressing was used. This was also kept moist with an oiled cloth covering. The continuous application of moist dressings was intended to prevent secretions from drying and forming a hard, painful crust over the wound, which, by retaining emissions, would cause great pain.[44] Of course, today this "painful crust" is recognized as a scab and considered a necessary part of the healing process.

Surgeons were able occasionally to observe the advantages of exposing wounds to the air and dry dressings. Purely by accident, the Confederate wounded taken to Williamsport, Maryland, after the Battle of Gettysburg were not treated for several days. Their wounds were exposed to the air, which, as previously noted, was thought to be detrimental. Yet, according to one account, these men healed favorably. Cases in which soldiers packed their own wounds with sawdust or bandaged them with clothing, or in which maggots ate the infected and dying tissue, offered quite remarkable results. The military surgeons, however, viewed such outcomes as aberrations and not the results of the exclusion of standard treatments. Moist dressings remained the prescribed treatment for the duration of the war.

37. Chisolm, *Manual of Military Surgery*, 215.
38. Kuz and Bengston, *Orthopaedic Injuries*, 15.
39. Cunningham, *Doctors in Gray*, 232.
40. Kuz and Bengston, *Orthopaedic Injuries*, 16.
41. Chisolm, *Manual of Military Surgery*, 192.
42. Cunningham, *Doctors in Gray*, 232.
43. Chisolm, *Manual of Military Surgery*, 192-193.
44. Chisolm, *Manual of Military Surgery*, 200.

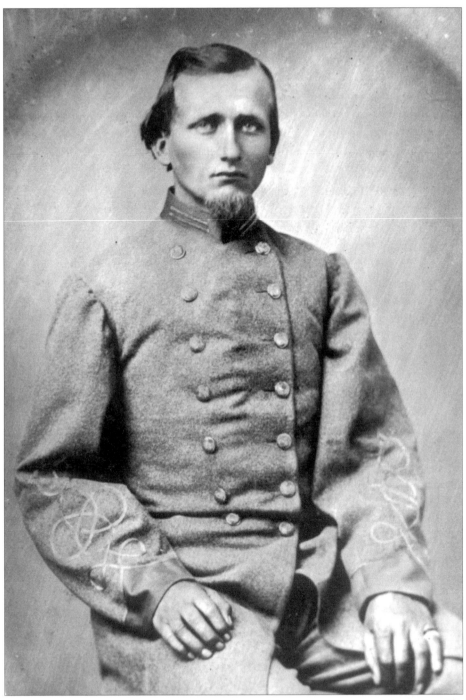

Henry Clay Koonce, a farmer in Jones County, enlisted on April 29, 1862, at age nineteen. He served as a first lieutenant in Company K, Sixty-first North Carolina Troops. On September 30, 1864, Koonce was wounded in an unsuccessful attempt to recapture Fort Harrison in the Richmond defenses. As a result of his wound, he lost his lower left leg. An invoice, dated November 15, 1866, indicates that he received a Jewett artificial leg from the state. He appears to have been living in Lenoir County at that time, but by 1870, he had returned to Jones County and his life as a farmer. Image courtesy of Lucien M. Koonce.

Because the benefits of antiseptics and disinfectants were not yet widely recognized, post-surgical infections were devastating. Gangrene, tetanus, blood poisoning, and erysipelas, an infection in the streptococcus family, were the most common and deadly. While some hospitals experimented with facility-wide treatments and preventative measures, infections were usually treated with local applications of charcoal, meal poultices, or cloth dipped in turpentine.[45] When topical treatments failed, doctors often simply tried to make their patients comfortable by administering alcohol and opiates.[46] Chisolm even recommended that tetanus patients, if able, be permitted the "constant smoking of strong cigars" to calm the spasms.[47] These treatments, of course, had limited and varied success. That the amputees survived the surgery and resulting infections under the conditions that existed during the Civil War is, indeed, a testament to the human body's ability to heal itself.

Rehabilitation of the Amputee

Amputees have always had to face a variety of physical and psychological challenges during rehabilitation. In reality, it is difficult to separate the physical from the psychological impediments. Even purely physical activities, such as walking, dancing, and completing everyday chores, provide psychological gratification that is scarcely noticed until such activities are curtailed. People value being physically independent and able, and are emotionally devastated by the loss of such independence.

The amputee must also adjust to the change in his outward appearance and how others respond to him. A suitable artificial limb helps the amputee to be less conspicuous and to avoid unwanted attention. While an artificial arm will not provide a firm handshake, nor will an artificial leg eliminate a limp, prosthetic devices do enable an amputee to resume a more routine life-style. The patient's acceptance and successful use of an artificial limb is the first, and most important, step in the psychological healing process.[48]

Certainly, the use of an artificial limb does not ensure rapid rehabilitation and, in fact, often causes the wearer a great deal of pain and discomfort. The standard complaints about prosthetic devices are skin irritation, excessive heat and perspiration, unusual sensations in the stump, fatigue, and difficulty in controlling movements. Arm amputees are much less tolerant of these troubles. The artificial arm

---

45. Kuz and Bengston, *Orthopaedic Injuries*, 16; Chisolm, *Manual of Military Surgery*, 243.

46. J. F. Shaffner Sr. to my dear friends, August 5, 1862, Shaffner Diary and Papers, Private Collections, State Archives.

47. Chisolm, *Manual of Military Surgery*, 265.

48. Sidney Fishman, "Amputation," in *Psychological Practices with the Physically Disabled*, ed. James F. Garrett and Edna S. Levine (New York: Columbia University Press, 1962), 7.

does not perform the crucial function of the leg and pulls on the amputee's stump rather than supporting it.[49] In regard to Civil War amputees, one must also consider that the stumps produced by the surgical procedures of the time often were not conducive to the use of artificial limbs. Protruding bones, or those left close to the skin's surface, and ragged scar tissue caused pain and frustration for amputees trying to use prostheses.

Another obstacle faced by amputees was phantom pain, that mysterious pain that seems to come from a missing limb. It was not only uncomfortable but also disconcerting. Though varying in degree and duration, phantom pain is experienced by virtually all amputees, particularly during the early stages of recovery. Raw nerve endings send signals to the brain that are misconstrued, and pain is assigned to a limb that no longer exists. A good example of how the brain can misinterpret signals is the headache that occasionally follows the eating of cold foods. The nerves in the roof of the mouth are along the same pathway as those in the forehead; the brain sometimes misreads signals from the roof of the mouth and transmits the pain to the forehead. Similarly, pain in the stump may be assigned to the amputated region by the brain, as the pathway of the nerves has been interrupted. Regardless of the scientific explanation, this painful specter of the amputee's missing limb often hinders rehabilitation. Some amputees are driven to alcoholism and drug abuse in an effort to reduce awareness of the phantom pain.[50] Many Civil War amputees, who were given alcohol and opiates while in the hospital, sought comfort in them after the war. Psychological healing, strength, and confidence are crucial to keep amputees from turning to such self-destructive, temporary solutions. In addition, with proper adjustment, phantom pain frequently decreases over time.

Artificial Limbs for North Carolina's Confederate Veterans

Confederate amputees, trying to regain a semblance of their former lives, found postwar southern society to be suffering from its own form of phantom pain. Slavery no longer existed, the economy had collapsed, the Confederacy was abolished, and many fathers, husbands, and sons were dead. In the war's aftermath, Confederate memorial movements, such as the Ladies Memorial Associations, were established throughout the South to honor the dead and their cause. "Organized bereavement," as one author has termed it, emphasized the loss of life and the end of a way of life.[51] While these memorial movements focused on glorifying the dead, they did little to improve conditions for the living amputees. The impoverished, mangled survivors, as reminders of the true horrors of the fight for the "lost cause," countered the idealistic

49. Friedman, "Amputation," 69.
50. Barja and Sherman, *What to Expect*, 20-21, 23.
51. Gaines M. Foster, *Ghosts of the Confederacy* (New York: Oxford University Press, 1987), 47.

image propagated by the memorialists. Arguably, the romantic idealization inherent in these groups detracted attention from and delayed addressing the practical, pressing needs of the amputees.

The Federal government and a Confederate association had initiated programs to provide amputees with limbs during the war.[52] The Association to Purchase Artificial Limbs for Maimed Soldiers began in the Confederacy in early 1864. Despite economic hardships in the South, the association collected approximately fifty thousand dollars within a matter of days.[53] Beginning in 1862, the Federal government provided money to Union amputees to purchase artificial limbs. The allowances were fifty dollars for an arm and seventy-five dollars for a leg. Commissioned officers, however, were not given this allowance until 1868. Furthermore, an 1866 act of Congress provided transportation for Union amputees to and from fittings for their prostheses, while legislation in 1870 furnished replacement limbs every five years.[54]

North Carolina rapidly responded to the needs of its Confederate amputees. The General Assembly passed a resolution on January 23, 1866, asking Gov. Jonathan Worth "to make a contract with some manufacturer of artificial limbs to supply the need of the State at an early day." In explanation, the resolution states: "And, whereas it is considered an eminent work of charity and of justice to assist all [who lost their limbs in service to the State of North Carolina] with the common funds of the State to procure necessary limbs, and thus to restore them, as far as practicable, to the comfortable use of their persons, to the enjoyment of life and to the ability to earn a subsistence."[55]

An editorial that appeared in Raleigh's *Daily Standard*, on January 19, 1866, the day on which this resolution was introduced, mentions the Federal program for supplying limbs and encourages support for a similar program in North Carolina to serve Confederate veterans. The writer claims that the legs would "make the man almost over again" and allow him to become a "producer" rather than a "consumer."[56] Interestingly, the *Standard* was the Unionist newspaper, and while its support for the artificial-limbs program was economically based, it was nonetheless support. The following day the pro-Confederate *Raleigh Sentinel* included an article declaring that the resolution was "a timely and eminently proper movement" and that "the State owes them, at least, this small token of her appreciation . . . prompted by humane and

---

52. Laurann Figg, "Clothing Adaptations of Civil War Amputees" (master's thesis, Iowa State University, 1990), 14; "Association to Purchase Artificial Limbs for Maimed Soldiers," *Confederate States Medical and Surgical Journal* 1 (April 1864): 59.

53. "Association to Purchase Artificial Limbs for Maimed Soldiers," 59.

54. Figg, "Clothing Adaptations of Civil War Amputees," 15.

55. Resolution of January 23, 1866, Resolutions, General Assembly Session Records, State Archives.

56. *Daily Standard* (Raleigh), January 19, 1866.

honorable motives."[57] Nowhere can any opposition to this resolution be found. The *Standard* writer went so far as to state that "no act could be passed which would be more acceptable to our people. They will cheerfully pay the small amount of taxes necessary to effect this object."[58]

In response to the mandate, Governor Worth advised the General Assembly in a letter of February 12, 1866, that he would ask each county sheriff to "ascertain and inform [him] how many limbs will be required for his county, distinguishing the number of legs, from the number of arms."[59] Worth speculated that more arm amputees would be reported because soldiers' legs were protected by breastworks and leg amputations were more likely to cause fatal complications. According to the numerous sheriffs' lists in the State Archives, slightly more missing arms were reported than legs.[60]

By the time of his letter to the General Assembly, Worth had concluded from correspondence with artificial-limb manufacturers that even the best prosthetic arms were primarily ornamental and not particularly functional. Preliminary reports from the counties and the governor's conclusions likely led to the assembly's amended resolution of February 15, 1866, which practically reiterated a portion of Worth's letter. This revision provided only artificial legs at no charge and commutations of seventy dollars to amputees who wished to procure their own choice of leg or did not want one. Arms could be purchased through the state for fifty dollars.[61] This policy was changed exactly one year later when the General Assembly approved a resolution to provide artificial arms or commutations of fifty dollars.[62] Perhaps letters such as that written by E. G. Cranford in December 1866 helped to sway the lawmakers. Cranford, who had been wounded at Spotsylvania Court House, reported that he was disabled from the loss of his "lift" arm, but that if he were given an artificial arm, he could "git to bisness." Furthermore, he argued, "It would be bad for a man to fight four years for his country and loose an arm and then have to pay for a wooden arm."[63]

In an interesting aside, the legislature, during the debate on purchasing limbs, considered an amendment to provide artificial limbs for women. While politically correct by today's standards, the amendment is mysterious in that no woman who fought for North Carolina reported having lost a limb. After some debate, the

---

57. *Raleigh Sentinel,* January 20, 1866.

58. *Daily Standard,* January 19, 1866.

59. Jonathan Worth to General Assembly, February 12, 1866, Jonathan Worth, Governors Letter Books, State Archives.

60. Sheriffs' Lists in Correspondence Relating to Artificial Limbs, 1866-1869, Civil War Collection, Military Collection, State Archives, and Jonathan Worth, Governors Papers, 1866, State Archives.

61. Resolution of February 15, 1866, Resolutions, General Assembly Session Records, State Archives.

62. Resolution of February 15, 1867, Resolutions, General Assembly Session Records, State Archives.

63. E. G. Cranford to Jonathan Worth, December 7, 1866, Jonathan Worth, Governors Papers, State Archives.

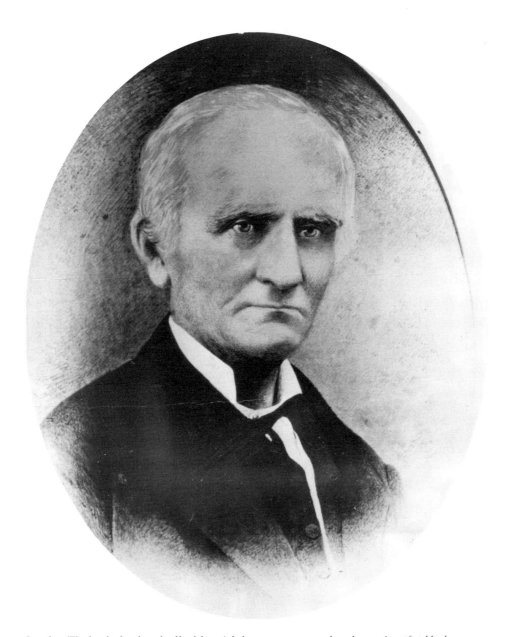

Jonathan Worth, who lived much of his life in Asheboro, was governor when the state's artificial limbs program began in 1866. The General Assembly authorized Worth to contract with an artificial limbs manufacturer, and after considering several options, he selected the Jewett's Patent Leg Company. Image courtesy of State Archives.

Executive Office,

RALEIGH, N. C. FEB. 5TH, 1866.

To the Sheriff of Harnett County,

Sir :

The General Assembly has ordered me to supply an artificial limb to every soldier who lost his limb in the service of the State in the late war, which I understand is intended to embrace every citizen of the State who lost an arm or leg while in the military service of the Confederate or State Government. It is necessary that I should know how many are to be supplied. I ask you in behalf of those maimed men, to report to me at an early day, how many such soldiers are in your county, distinguishing those who have lost a leg from those who have lost an arm.

Jonathan Worth,

Gov. of N. C.

During the planning phase of the state's artificial limbs program, Governor Worth asked sheriffs around the state to determine the number of limbs that would be needed in their county. This is a copy of the request sent to the sheriff of Harnett County. Jonathan Worth, Governors Papers, State Archives.

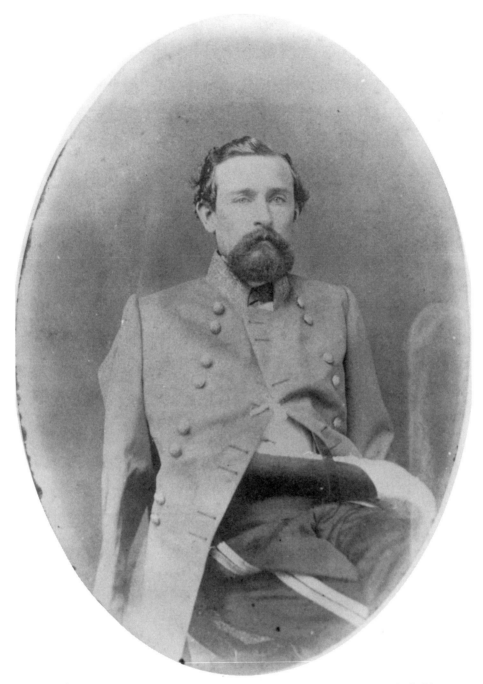

North Carolina expanded its artificial limbs program in February 1867 to include veterans who had lost an arm. Amputees could choose an artificial arm or a fifty-dollar commutation. Brig. Gen. Laurence S. Baker lost the use of his arm after being wounded near Brandy Station, Virginia, on July 31, 1863. Though his arm was not amputated, he was still eligible to receive fifty dollars from the state. Baker, a West Point graduate, had been a career military officer before the war. His damaged arm, however, forced him to find a new vocation. After trying several jobs in North Carolina and Virginia, he became a railroad agent for the Seaboard Air Line in Suffolk, Virginia. Image courtesy of State Archives.

proposal was referred to a joint committee, then tabled, at the committee's recommendation, on January 21, 1866.[64]

In a letter to the General Assembly in February 1866, Worth expressed support for a contract with Jewett's Patent Leg Company of Washington, D.C., because "a young man of good character and skilled as a mechanic in the manufacture of artificial limbs and a native of this state was working in the establishment."[65] Silas M. Stone of Franklin County had written to Worth in January about John T. Ball, a native North Carolinian and "master Leg maker" who wanted to return home. Ball had previously made harnesses and cabinets in New Bern. Stone, a veteran of the Fifty-fifth North Carolina, had lost a leg after being wounded at Gettysburg. He had purchased an artificial leg from Jewett's in 1865 for one hundred dollars. Pleased with the leg and the work of Ball, Stone proposed a plan to bring the craftsman back to North Carolina to oversee the manufacture of artificial limbs.[66]

In a letter to Governor Worth dated March 8, 1866, A. H. St. John of Jewett's Patent Leg Company offered North Carolina two contract options. The first would have allowed North Carolina to buy exclusive rights to the leg by purchasing two patents for twelve thousand dollars. The patents, numbers 16,360 and 29,494, were issued to Benjamin W. Jewett of Gilford, New Hampshire, in 1857 and 1860, respectively. In addition, Jewett's would furnish the wooden blocks, springs, and joints needed to manufacture the legs for ten dollars a set. The second option required that the state provide Jewett's with a building in North Carolina where limbs could be manufactured and pay a five-thousand-dollar advance. Jewett's would then sell legs to the state for seventy-five dollars each.[67] Worth opted for the latter plan, keeping open for one month the option to purchase the patents. The April 19, 1866, contract adjusted the cost of each leg from seventy-five to seventy dollars.[68] There is no evidence that the state ever purchased the patent.

The building provided to Jewett's was in Raleigh, but the exact location is unknown. Governor Worth, however, described the likely site in an April 19, 1866, letter, in which he asks if the state may occupy a building "in the north part of the

64. *Journal of the Senate of the General Assembly of the State of North Carolina at its Session of 1866-'67* (Raleigh: William E. Pell, 1867), 317.

65. Jonathan Worth to General Assembly, February 12, 1866, Governors Letter Books, State Archives.

66. Silas M. Stone to Gov. Jonathan Worth, January 25, 1866, Governors Papers, Governor Jonathan Worth, State Archives. Various records, including death certificates, Bible records, and city directories, indicate that Ball moved his family to Raleigh in 1866 and remained indefinitely.

67. A. H. St. John to Jonathan Worth, March 6, 1866, Correspondence Relating to Artificial Limbs, 1866-1869, Civil War Collection, State Archives.

68. Contract signed by Jonathan Worth and A. H. St. John, April 19, 1866, on back of letter from St. John to Worth, March 6, 1866, Correspondence Relating to Artificial Limbs, 1866-1869, Civil War Collection, State Archives.

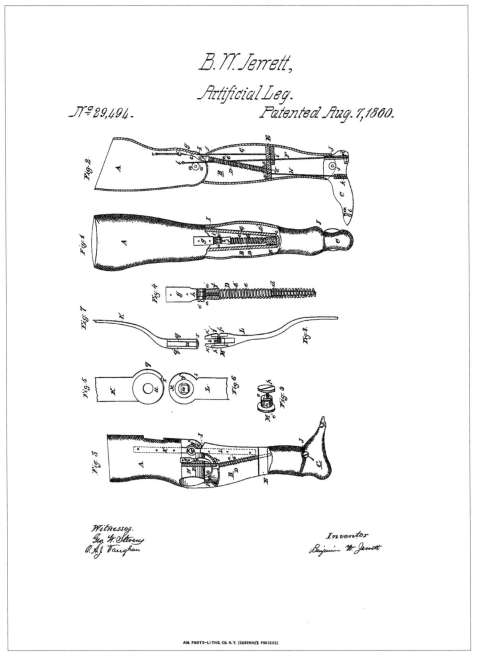

The Jewett's Patent Leg, seen in the patent sketch above (U.S. Patent number 29,494), was heralded for its "mechanical perfection" and the ease with which the wearer could complete basic repairs. Gov. Jonathan Worth contracted with the Jewett Company to provide artificial legs in March 1866. The company sent John T. Ball, a New Bern native and "master leg maker," to Raleigh, where he made limbs for North Carolina veterans until June 18, 1867. United States Patent and Trademark Office, Publication Number: 00029494, Section: Drawings (http://www.uspto.gov/patft/index.html), July 19, 2004.

city," which was "used—perhaps erected, for the manufacture of bayonets."[69] The Raleigh bayonet factory was conveniently located near the shops, and therefore the terminus, of the Raleigh and Gaston Railroad, near the junction of North and McDowell Streets.[70] Once the facility was in operation, the amputees were notified as to when they should report to Raleigh for fittings. Details of the program appeared in newspapers throughout the state, including the requirement that amputees obtain a certificate from the county clerk of court indicating their company, regiment, and which limb they had lost. Forms for this purpose were sent to all counties. Once the certificate was approved by the Artificial Limb Department, a component of the office of the State Adjutant General, the amputee would receive further instructions.[71]

Whether in imitation of the Federal artificial-limbs program or in response to pleas from maimed veterans, North Carolina devised a plan by which the amputees incurred no out-of-pocket expenses while in Raleigh. In addition, the state issued railroad passes for the trip to and from the capital. The fittings and adjustments usually took a couple of days, and a house was provided for the amputees during this time. The governor advised the amputees to bring blankets for bedding and a basket of bread and dried meat for their meals.[72]

In order to be considered for a commutation, disabled veterans were often required to travel to Raleigh to be examined by E. Burke Haywood, a former Confederate surgeon from Raleigh. Haywood was a graduate of the University of Pennsylvania Medical School, and during the war he had served as president of the North Carolina Board of Surgeons and the Confederate Army Medical Board. In a letter to Worth dated June 19, 1867, Haywood urged the governor to broaden the definition of "useless" limbs because the stringent interpretation then in effect, which required complete paralysis, prevented certification of deserving men to receive their commutations.[73]

The degree of satisfaction among recipients of North Carolina's artificial limbs varied widely. As human nature dictates, letters of complaint are more likely to be written than those expressing praise. Thus there are more letters from dissatisfied veterans, requesting new limbs or, more commonly, petitioning for the commutation in exchange for the return of a limb, than from those who were pleased. The general consensus among the discontented was that their stump was not conducive to the use

---

69. Jonathan Worth to Thomas H. Ruger, April 19, 1866, Jonathan Worth, Governors Papers, State Archives.

70. Elizabeth Reid Murray, *Wake, Capital County of North Carolina* (Raleigh: Capital County, 1983), 468.

71. Correspondence Relating to Artificial Limbs, 1866-1869, Civil War Collection, State Archives.

72. S. G. Ryan to Sheriff of Granville County, June 15, 1866, and S. G. Ryan to S. J. Carver, Sheriff of Beaufort County, June 15, 1866, Adjutant Generals Records, Letter Book of the Superintendent of the Department of Artificial Limbs, State Archives. See also Clyde Olin Fisher, "A Brief History of Confederate Pensions and Soldiers' Relief in North Carolina" (master's thesis, Columbia University, 1916).

73. E. Burke Haywood to Jonathan Worth, Jonathan Worth, Governors Papers, State Archives.

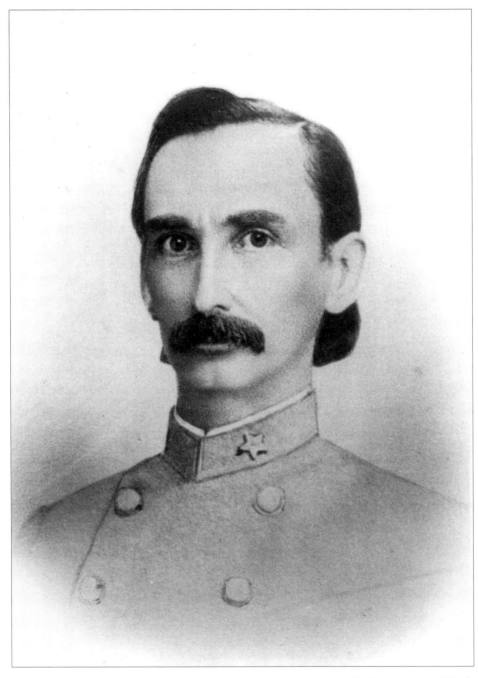

To qualify for a commutation, disabled veterans had to be examined by Edmund Burke Haywood in Raleigh. Trained at the University of Pennsylvania Medical School, Haywood had been a Confederate army surgeon and supervisor of Raleigh's military hospitals. After the war, he was head of the state Board of Public Charities and surgery chairman of the North Carolina Board of Medical Examiners. Image courtesy of State Archives.

of an artificial limb. Amputees complained of pain, difficulty of movement, and problems with the operation of their apparatus. J. L. Cathey of Asheville, who had lost his right leg after being wounded at Chickamauga, said that while he could walk on the leg in the shop in Raleigh, once he got home he could not walk on the uneven ground outside. He went on to say, "I have worn it one time and since that time I cannot get my leg in it to try it anymore[.] my stump is to short for a Leg of the fashion mine is."[74] Similar comments were made about artificial arms. J. M. McLean, who lost his right arm as a result of a wound received at Gettysburg, wrote: "I can say that the arm is really of no service to me, except to fill the vacancy. It is an incumbrance & hurts me to wear it. The money would be of more service to me than the arm."[75]

There were, of course, some expressions of appreciation, such as that from Pinkney M. Amos, who had served in the Forty-fifth Regiment North Carolina Troops and had lost his left leg after being wounded during Jubal Early's Maryland campaign in the summer of 1864.[76] Amos wrote, "I have used my leg sucksessfuly & worne out the straps So that I must have new."[77] B. F. Fonville wrote one of the few extant letters praising the artificial arm: "I am well pleased with it[.] I can use it in riding or hold my paper in wrighting or holding any thing that is not to heavy it is of a good deal of servis to a man that [is obliged] to use one[.] I would not be without it for what I had to pay for it."[78] Fonville evidently purchased an arm for fifty dollars before the state began to provide them. W. R. Ferguson stated that he utilized his artificial leg with the help of a cane but complained that "it makes so much fuss any one can [hear] it be fore I get in a hundred yards."[79]

Ferguson was apparently aware of the relative ease with which the leg could be repaired, for he asked the Artificial Limb Department for "2 ½ yards of Indian-rubber & 24 small brass screws" and directions as to how to oil the joint.[80] Fixing the leg was

74. J. L. Cathey to S. G. Ryan, February 22, 1867, Correspondence Relating to Artificial Limbs, 1866-1869, Civil War Collection, State Archives; Louis H. Manarin and Weymouth T. Jordan Jr., comps., *North Carolina Troops, 1861-1865: A Roster*, 15 vols. to date (Raleigh: Division of Archives and History, Department of Cultural Resources, 1966-), 14:576; Walter Clark, ed., *Histories of the Several Regiments and Battalions from North Carolina in the Great War, 1861-'65*, 5 vols. (Raleigh and Goldsboro: State of North Carolina, 1901), 3:488.

75. J. M. McLean to S. G. Ryan, February 23, 1867, Correspondence Relating to Artificial Limbs, 1866-1869, Civil War Collection, State Archives; Manarin and Jordan, *North Carolina Troops*, 6:644.

76. Manarin and Jordan, *North Carolina Troops*, 11:46.

77. Pinkney M. Amos to S. G. Ryan, March 17, 1868, Correspondence Relating to Artificial Limbs, 1866-1869, Civil War Collection, State Archives.

78. B. F. Fonville to S. G. Ryan, March 4, 1867, Correspondence Relating to Artificial Limbs, 1866-1869, Civil War Collection, State Archives.

79. W. R. Ferguson to S. G. Ryan, November 2, 1866, Correspondence Relating to Artificial Limbs, 1866-1869, Civil War Collection, State Archives.

80. W. R. Ferguson to S. G. Ryan, November 2, 1866, Correspondence Relating to Artificial Limbs, 1866-1869, Civil War Collection, State Archives.

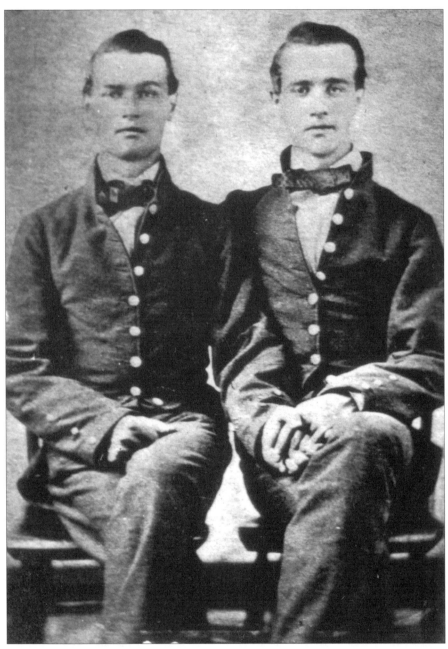

Brothers Levi J. and Henry J. Walker of Mecklenburg County served in Company B, Thirteenth North Carolina Troops, and each lost his left leg as a result of wounds. Levi, the younger brother and a private, was wounded while carrying the colors during an assault on Cemetery Hill at Gettysburg on July 1, 1863. Doctors at a field hospital amputated his leg, and he was subsequently taken prisoner. Henry, a third lieutenant, was wounded near Hagerstown, Maryland, as Lee's army retreated after the defeat at Gettysburg, and he too was taken prisoner. After

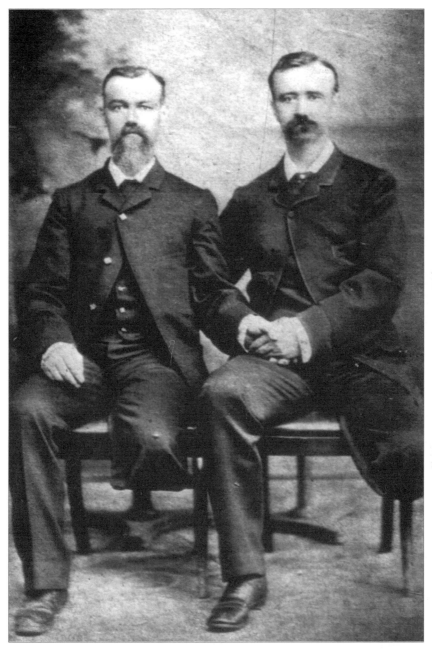

the war the brothers returned to Charlotte and conducted successful careers—Henry as a doctor and Levi as a merchant. Levi married after the war. Just before the wedding, however, he fell and broke his artificial leg. Henry allowed Levi to use his prosthesis so that he could stand during the ceremony. Photographs from Walter Clark, ed., *Histories of the Several Regiments and Battalions from North Carolina in the Great War, 1861-'65*, vol. 4 (Raleigh and Goldsboro: State of North Carolina, 1901), facing 405.

so easy that even such requests for spare parts and instructions were rare. The Jewett's Patent Leg was known, and in part selected, for its simple repairs.

The facility operated by Jewett's Patent Leg Company in Raleigh, where the state's artificial arms were also manufactured, remained open until June 18, 1867. At that time, A. H. St. John reported to Governor Worth that the shop no longer had enough work to continue on-site manufacturing. St. John promised that Ball would remain in Raleigh to complete repairs and make new limbs. Repairs would be made for free if the defect was the manufacturer's fault. Problems caused by ordinary wear were not covered, however. It seems that only two legs were ever returned because of faulty workmanship.[81] As previously mentioned, the condition of some amputees' stumps made the use of artificial limbs difficult. If men with this problem waived their commutation and tried to use a limb, only to find that they could not, the prosthesis could be exchanged for money. In the case of a leg, the amount was fifty dollars. No figure has been found for the return of an arm.[82]

In keeping with the legislature's aim to help amputees reestablish themselves financially, a bill was proposed on February 13, 1867, providing, "That any Person who lost a Leg or an arm in the military Service of the late Confederate States, Shall be allowed a License to retail Spiritous Liquors by a measure less than a Quart without paying any Tax for Such License, State or County . . . [or] any Tax State or County."[83] This measure reflected the widely held belief that the state should help amputees resume productive lives, even to the point of finding a livelihood for them. John C. Gorman of Raleigh, in a letter to the governor dated February 26, 1867, expressed support for the proposal and offered a candidate for the new program, A. C. Christmas, an amputee from Wilson County. Gorman explained that Christmas could not use his right arm because of a wound received at Spotsylvania Court House and that he was a man "of steady habits and of upright character."[84] The bill, however, was tabled the very day Gorman penned his letter. Whether the measure's demise was caused by a general disapproval of liquor or the fear that some veterans might seek solace in their merchandise, the amputees were forced to find other employment.

According to monthly entries in the state treasurer's cash book, the total cost of the artificial-limbs program to the state from 1865 to 1871 was $81,310.12.[85] A review of the auditor's records and treasurer's journal for the same period confirms this total. The first two years of the program were the most expensive, with $22,656.29 spent in

81. A. H. St. John to Jonathan Worth, June 18, 1867, Correspondence Relating to Artificial Limbs, 1866-1869, Civil War Collection, State Archives; Silas M. Stone to Jonathan Worth, January 25, 1866, Jonathan Worth, Governors Papers, State Archives.

82. Correspondence Relating to Artificial Limbs, 1866-1869, Civil War Collection, State Archives.

83. House Bill 354, General Assembly Session Records, January-March 1867, State Archives.

84. John C. Gorman to Jonathan Worth, February 26, 1867, Jonathan Worth Papers, Private Collections, State Archives.

85. Treasurer's Cash Book 4, 1865-1871, Treasurer's and Comptroller's Papers, State Archives.

1866 and $54,403.83 in 1867. By 1868, the total was only $3,470. That fell to $150 in 1870, and by 1871, there were no reported expenses.[86]

Comparing North Carolina's program and expenses with those of other states is difficult because few states have organized records pertaining to artificial limbs. South Carolina is an exception. The South Carolina legislature voted to provide artificial legs in September 1866, and tax collectors were instructed to compile lists of amputees in their districts. The General Assembly, after considering these lists, allocated a lump sum of twenty thousand dollars for artificial limbs in November of that year. South Carolina selected the Bly leg for their amputees and contributed $74.65 per leg. The program was stopped in 1869, but revived in 1877 and included artificial arms.[87]

Virginia's legislature appropriated twenty thousand dollars to purchase artificial limbs and to establish the Board of Commissioners on Artificial Limbs on January 29, 1867.[88] Their procedures were similar to North Carolina's, and, in fact, W. B. Watkins, head of Virginia's Artificial Limbs Board, wrote Governor Worth on February 12, 1867, thanking him for his "valuable suggestions" and stating that they would be "of much help in carrying out and consummating the purposes of our General Assembly."[89] Although Virginia offered to replace limbs after five years, the state did not provide commutations to those unable to use limbs until 1882. Bounties for the exchange of unusable limbs were not offered until 1872.[90]

Mississippi seems to have been second among the Confederate states, after North Carolina, in establishing an artificial-limbs program. The Mississippi legislature passed a resolution on October 25, 1866, providing limbs or commutations for both arms and legs, and allotting thirty thousand dollars for the project. Their artificial limbs department produced an extraordinary "Report of Maimed State and Confederate Soldiers" that was published in the House Journal of 1866-1867. This report provides the name, rank, company, and regiment of each soldier in the program; how and by what the soldier was maimed; when and where he was wounded; and even what type of operation was performed.[91]

On February 2, 1867, the Arkansas legislature appropriated ten thousand dollars for the fiscal year for artificial limbs. A list was to be compiled by the local tax

86. Treasurer's Cash Book 4, 1865-1871, Treasurer's and Comptroller's Papers, State Archives.

87. Patrick J. McCawley, *Artificial Limbs for Confederate Soldiers* (Columbia: South Carolina Department of Archives and History, 1992), 1-2.

88. Jennifer Davis McDaid, "With Lame Legs and No Money," *Virginia Cavalcade* (winter 1998): 16.

89. W. B. Watkins to Jonathan Worth, February 12, 1867, Jonathan Worth, Governors Papers, State Archives.

90. McDaid, "With Lame Legs and No Money," 18-19.

91. State of Mississippi, *Journal of the House of Representatives of the State of Mississippi* (Jackson: J. J. Shannon and Company, 1866), 99-101, 132-160.

assessors, and special taxes were to be levied "if necessary" for the limbs and the "general support of maimed and indigent."[92]

The remarkably detailed legislative journals of Texas provide an exceptional account of the financial constraints and civic loyalties that must have affected the artificial-limbs debates in all of the former Confederate states. The Texas House of Representatives appropriated fifty thousand dollars on August 10, 1866, to buy "Artificial or cork legs" for Confederate veterans. The resolution to this effect was sent to the Committee on Finance, which reported on September 20 that, after having given the matter "more than *ordinary consideration* and with much *reluctance* [we] have arrived at the conclusion that owing to our present financial embarrassments, as well as the great difficulties attending the execution of the project, therefore it would be impolitic to make the appropriation referred to."

The Texas House asked the committee to continue to investigate the best means by which the state could institute a program for distributing legs. In October, a Mr. Foster of the House of Representatives introduced a joint resolution suggesting that each member of the legislature deposit one hundred dollars with the governor to be used for purchasing legs for maimed veterans. This resolution, too, was referred to the Committee on Finance. Four days later the committee reported that they would allocate a total of one hundred dollars to the governor. This money was to be used for postage and other expenses incurred in gathering information from artificial-limb companies, which might be used later for a program to purchase and distribute cork legs. The legislature vowed to resume the quest during the next session, which was to be held in 1870.[93] There is no mention, however, in that year's House and Senate journals of an artificial-limbs program.

While the state of Louisiana did not provide artificial limbs in the seven years following the Civil War, the Ladies Benevolent Association did furnish them in 1866.[94] Interestingly, the General Assembly of 1873 addressed the needs of the veterans and widows of the War of 1812. This delayed recognition, and the attitude it implies, perhaps helps to explain the lack of legislation to aid the Confederate wounded. Georgia did not provide any artificial limbs for the state's Confederate amputees until 1877.[95] The Confederate states that did not adequately aid their maimed veterans were not indifferent; they were limited in what they could do by the constrictions of Reconstruction and a lack of funds.

92. State of Arkansas, *Acts of the General Assembly of the State of Arkansas* (Little Rock: Woodruff and Blocher, 1867), 90, 95.

93. State of Texas, *Journal of the House of Representatives of the Eleventh Legislature* (Austin: State Gazette, 1866), 29, 338, 728, 785.

94. David M. Camp, *The American Yearbook and National Register for 1869* (Hartford: O. D. Case and Company, 1869), 350.

95. State of Georgia, *Acts and Resolutions of the General Assembly of the State of Georgia, 1878-1879* (Atlanta: Jas. P. Harrison, 1880), 41-42.

Unquestionably, North Carolina's artificial-limbs program faced similar problems, but with public and governmental support, the state persevered. Even the Reconstruction government continued the program established by its predecessors until amputees were provided with either limbs or commutations. The strong public sentiment that the veterans should be compensated carried the program to fruition despite the federal administration's disdain for Confederate veterans in general.

The phantom pain of the amputees and of a devastated society was meliorated in North Carolina by the artificial-limbs program. The program was a success in the wake of failure. After defeat, the loss of thousands of lives, and economic ruin, the state's citizens still had the ability to achieve something noble by repaying, to a degree, those who had literally risked life and limb.

Rarity in Red Springs:
Jewett Leg Preserved by Hanna Family

Since beginning my research on North Carolina's artificial-limbs program in 1997, I have viewed many records concerning Jewett's Patent Leg, the prosthesis that the state of North Carolina purchased for its veterans. An extant example of the limb, however, has been difficult to locate. Queries to numerous museums over the years failed to produce results. I, nevertheless, maintained hope that somewhere in private hands a Jewett leg might still exist. Every report I received about a North Carolina Confederate veteran's leg, however, led to either a peg leg or other homemade substitute, or in rare cases, a different brand of commercially produced prosthesis. Since, according to the records, the peg leg owners had received Jewett legs, it became clear that the Jewett legs were unlikely to have lasted through the wearer's lifetime, much less to the present.

In April 2003, Jason Tomberlin, then correspondence archivist with the North Carolina State Archives, received a request from Duncan Hanna of Red Springs, North Carolina, for a copy of the Confederate soldier's pension application filed by his grandfather, Robert Alexander Hanna. Tomberlin brought this request to my attention because it indicated that Hanna possessed an artificial leg that his grandfather had worn. Though disappointed before, I still had hope that this could be a rare example of the Jewett leg. I promptly wrote to Mr. Hanna expressing my interest in the leg and including my e-mail address. A few weeks later, I received an e-mail with no text except for the name "Duncan Hanna" and the notation that there were several attachments. What I saw in the attached pictures made my heart skip. The photographs not only closely resembled contemporary sketches of the Jewett Patent Leg, but one image in particular, of the sole of the foot, showed several distinctive features specified on those sketches.

To have additional photographs made, I arranged a meeting between Archives and History photographer Alan Westmoreland and Duncan Hanna. Ultimately, Hanna generously allowed Westmoreland to bring the leg to Raleigh so that photographs could be taken in the studio and so that I, and others, could examine the prosthesis closely. Len Hambleton, conservator at the North Carolina Museum of History, was so captivated with the artifact that he agreed to clean it and perform some repairs. His work helped make it possible for me to positively identify the leg as a Jewett's Patent Leg.

Duncan Hanna's grandfather, Robert Alexander Hanna, served in Company K of the Twenty-sixth North Carolina Troops. He enlisted in Anson County on July 1, 1861, and exactly two years later, at Gettysburg, was wounded in the head and left leg, just above the ankle. The leg wound suppurated for about a month before the amputation was performed, but fortunately the infection had not become systemic. Hanna first contacted the state to procure an artificial leg in June 1866, when he submitted a form to Gov. Jonathan Worth's office. The Jewett Patent Leg Company invoiced the state of North Carolina, which then paid for Hanna's leg in January 1867. Hanna, according to his grandson, usually saved the Jewett leg for special occasions and wore homemade prostheses while working on his farm. It was probably Hanna's prudence that insured the survival of the Jewett leg. Damage from wear to the bottom of the foot illustrates how these delicately made legs could wear out. Robert Alexander Hanna, who died in 1917 at about age eighty-five, had his Jewett leg for fifty years. That he kept and maintained it throughout his life is extraordinary, and that his descendants did the same is no less remarkable.

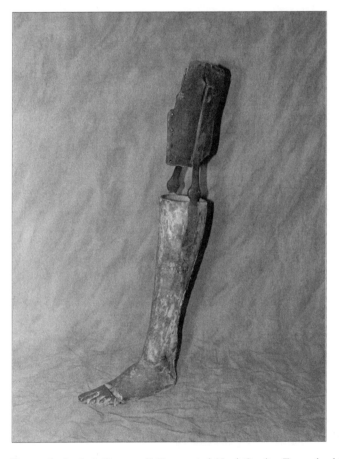

Robert Alexander Hanna, who fought in Company K, Twenty-sixth North Carolina Troops, lost his left leg after being wounded at Gettysburg on July 1, 1863. In 1867, the state gave him this artificial leg, crafted by Jewett's Patent Leg Company. Hanna's leg had been amputated below the knee, so his stump rested inside the base of the prosthetic limb, while the leather top laced around his thigh. So well-balanced is the leg that it is free standing in this photograph. Photograph by Alan Westmoreland.

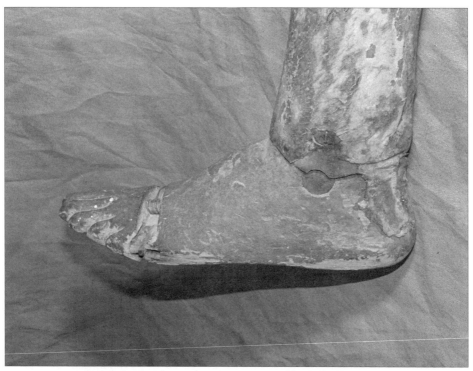

The foot of Hanna's prosthesis demonstrates the detailed craftsmanship of the Jewett leg. The spring that allowed the toe section to flex while walking is visible, in line with the second toe.

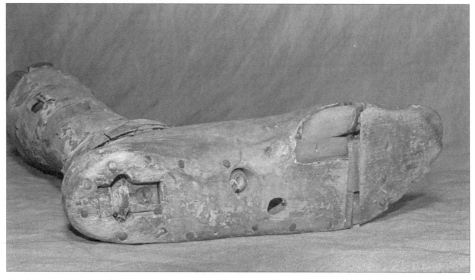

The bottom of the foot of Hanna's prosthesis shows where the pulleys that operated the leg connected at the heel and arch. North Carolina Museum of History conservator Len Hambleton filled the gap where the wood had splintered at the toe hinge. The foot probably was covered originally with a leather base, as suggested by the nails encircling the perimeter. Nevertheless, the delicate woodcarving appears to have worn down over time, a factor that helps to explain the rarity of the Jewett's Patent Leg today. Both photographs by Alan Westmoreland.

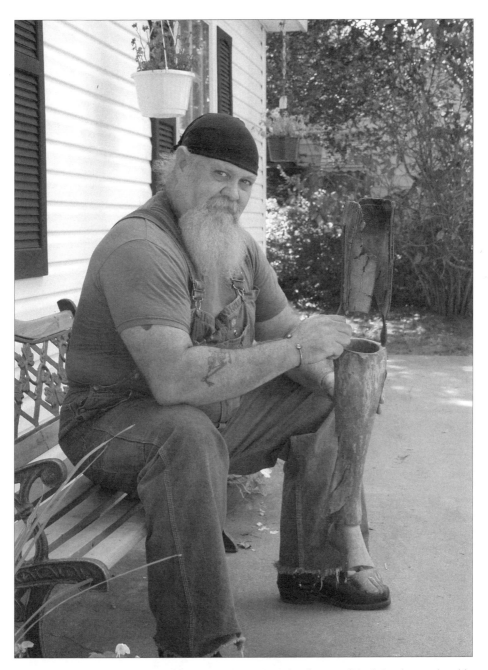

Duncan Hanna of Red Springs poses with the Jewett's Patent Leg that the state of North Carolina purchased for his grandfather in 1867. His grandfather, Robert Alexander Hanna, died in 1917, and the Hanna family preserved the leg. Duncan Hanna explained that his grandfather made peg legs to wear while working on the farm, saving the manufactured limb for special occasions. Photograph by Alan Westmoreland.

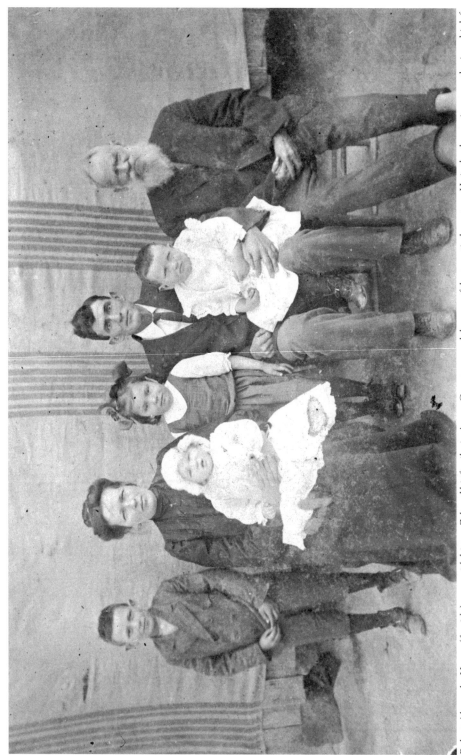

Robert Alexander Hanna (*far right*) poses with his son Zeb and his family, in Anson County around the turn of the twentieth century. He is clearly wearing a prosthesis on his left leg in the photo. Hanna died in 1917 at about age eighty-five. Image courtesy of the Hanna family.

Index to Records in the North Carolina State Archives Related to Artificial Limbs for Confederate Veterans

COMPILED BY ANSLEY HERRING WEGNER

The following is an index of state documents in the North Carolina State Archives related to Civil War amputees, artificial-limb recipients, and veterans who requested commutations because they were unable to use an artificial limb. The index is arranged alphabetically by the veteran's surname and includes basic information from the records. This may include the county from which the veteran is corresponding, his unit, the date or dates of each record, the limb lost, and the collection in which each record can be found. A blank cell indicates that the information could not be found. Each veteran's information is placed in six columns on facing pages. To ease reading across the pages, the same number is placed to the left of the veteran's record on both pages. A number after the veteran's name indicates the number of records found for that individual. When various spellings of a name were found in the records, an attempt was made to determine the correct spelling. The alternate spellings used in the documents are given in parentheses.

Details from sources other than those listed in the location column are placed in brackets. For example, some soldiers' units were identified using *Histories of the Several Regiments and Battalions from North Carolina in the Great War, 1861-'65*; *North Carolina Troops, 1861-1865: A Roster*; and *The Roster of Confederate Soldiers, 1861-1865*. Cavalry and artillery regiments bear, in addition to their identifying number, an NCT designation. Abbreviations used in the index include: NCT-North Carolina Troops; NCST-North Carolina State Troops; PC-Private Collections; and IG-Inspector General.

Information in the location column indicates where researchers can find the original records. The date of a document is given in the date column opposite the document's location. If no date is given, see the date listed for the document above. The number in parentheses indicates how many documents bear the same date. In a few cases a number appears after the document's location. This indicates how many documents pertaining to that soldier are in the collection and have the same date. In a few instances information about one soldier can be found in another soldier's records. Cross references are included in such cases, with an asterisk placed next to

the document with the appropriate date. Other cross references are given to aid
researchers who are unsure of the spelling of the object of their search.

Records may be viewed at the North Carolina State Archives during normal
hours of operation, or researchers may request to receive copies of documents
through the mail by contacting the correspondence archivist at the State Archives.
The location codes are as follows:

AG 58

This volume, an 1866 Letter Book from the superintendent of the Artificial
Limb Department, A. S. Ryan, is filed in the Adjutant General's papers. It is a
letterpress book, a primitive means of copying outgoing correspondence using
onionskin paper and water-soluble ink. Many of the pages are difficult to read because
of smeared ink and tattered paper. Most letters contain one of two messages that were
commonly sent to the veterans: "Owing to the want of joints your leg will not be
completed when expected, but will be ready for delivery eight or ten days after the
time promised," or "By coming here you can get your limb which is now complete."

When this book was used, the state supplied only legs free of charge. Consequently, a general reference to "limbs" in the letter book probably refers to legs.

Aud 6.1

This volume, called "Register of Artificial Limbs 1866-1870," includes the
veteran's name, county, and military unit; the specific limb amputated and in some
cases how much of the limb was lost; and remarks indicating whether an artificial
limb or commutation was issued and on what date.

Aud 6.113

This box of materials from the Auditor's Office Pension Bureau records contains
the same two types of applications for commutations found in the Military
Collection and the Governors Papers.

CW Mil 41 and Jewett Invoices

These records are in the Civil War Collection within the State Archives'
Military Collection. The Jewett's Patent Leg Company invoices, called Jewett
Invoices in the index, are in a box labeled simply as Box 41. They are arranged
chronologically, listing the date the limb was delivered, to whom, and the
recipient's military unit.

The letters and forms, designated in the index as CW Mil 41, are arranged
alphabetically in Boxes 41.1 through 41.5. Lists of maimed soldiers from the various
counties are at the back of Box 41.5. The lists are alphabetized by county and
designated in the index as "Co. List."

Worth 1 through Worth 8

This designation indicates that there is a letter, form, or list related to the veteran filed chronologically in Gov. Jonathan Worth's papers. Worth's papers include lists of soldiers by county. These are indicated as "Co. List" in the index. There is also a list of Greensboro troops, which is designated "City List" in the index. Undated materials are filed in Box 8, where there is a separate folder for the lists of maimed soldiers.

Holden 1

This designation indicates that there is a letter, form, or list related to the veteran filed chronologically in Gov. W. W. Holden's papers.

T&C Cash Bk 4 (TC $ Bk 4)

In the early years of the artificial-limbs program, there were too many recipients of limbs and commutations for the Treasurer's and Comptroller's Office to list them by name in their accounts. In the waning years, however, names were recorded. The amount of money by a person's name helps to determine how that money was spent. For example, fifty dollars by the name of a recipient of a leg indicates that the prosthesis could not be used and was returned for a commutation. This is the best source for determining whether an amputee later returned a limb for the commutation.

	Claimant	County	Confederate Unit
1	Adams, David B. (3)	Union	Co. F, 35th NCT
2	Adams, J. T., Capt. (4)	Lincoln	Co. K, 49th NCT
3	Adams, S. P.	Cleveland	
4	Adcock, J. C. (3)	Chatham	Co. G, 26th NCT
5	Agner, John F. (2)	Rowan	Co. B, 46th NCT
6	Alexander, D. S.	Mecklenburg	
7	Alexander, Thomas M.	Mecklenburg	Co. F, 58th NCT
8	Allen, C. N., Capt. (5) (also Nick)	Wake	Co. D, 30th NCT
9	Allen, David (5)	Robeson	Co. K, 40th NCT
10	Allen, Fulton C. (4)	Anson	Co. E, 11th NCT
11	Allen, James	Person	[Co. H, 24th NCT]
12	Allen, John (2)	Caswell	[Co. C, 13th NCT]
13	Allen, Larkin	Cleveland	Co. G, 49th NCT
14	Allison, J. M.	Cleveland	Co. H, 28th NCT

	Date	Limb	Location
1	17 Aug 1866 21 Aug 1866 22 Oct 1866	Leg	Worth 3, form Aud. 6.1, p. 2 Worth 3, Co. List
2	15 May 1866 22 May 1866 24 May 1866 13 June 1866	Leg	Worth 2, letter Worth 2, forms Jewett Invoices Aud. 6.1, p. 1
3	no date	Arm	Worth 8, Co. List
4	5 Dec 1866 21 March 1867 29 March 1867	Arm	Worth 4, Co. List CW Military 41 Aud. 6.1, p. 1
5	23 April 1866 15 March 1867	Arm	CW Mil, Co. List Aud. 6.1, p. 1
6	9 Nov 1866	Loin	Worth 4, Co. List
7	6 June 1867	Leg	Aud. 6.1, p. 1
8	9 June 1866 21 March 1867 13 April 1867 15 April 1867 no date	Arm	Worth 3, order CW Military 41 Jewett Invoices Aud. 6.1, p. 1 CW Mil, Co. List
9	2 July 1866 18 Aug 1866 10 Oct 1866 13 Nov 1866 (2)	Leg	Worth 3, form Worth 3, letter Worth 3, Co. List Jewett Invoices Aud. 6.1, p. 1
10	9 June 1866 11 Dec 1866 19 Dec 1866 (2)	Leg	Worth 3, form CW Military 41 Jewett Invoices Aud. 6.1, p. 1
11	27 Nov 1866	Arm	Worth 4, Co. List
12	20 Feb 1866 14 Feb 1867	Leg	Worth 1, Co. List CW Military 41
13	6 April 1867	Arm	Aud. 6.1, p.1
14	8 April 1867	Arm	Aud. 6.1, p. 1

	Claimant	County	Confederate Unit
1	Allman, William C. (2) (also Allmond)	Stanly	Co. F, 5th NCST
2	Allred, John B. (2) (also Aldred)	Caswell	Co. H, 6th NCST
3	Almond, Green	Stanly	[Co. H, 14th NCT]
4	Alphin, Jesse J. (3) (also McAlphin)	Duplin	Co. I, 9th NCST (1st NC Cav.)
5	Amos, Pinkney M. (8) (also D. M. Amos)	Rockingham	Co. D, 45th NCT
6	Anderson, Creed R. (2)	McDowell and Burke	Co. E, 6th NCST
7	Anderson, G. A.	Mecklenburg	
8	Andrews, James	Alamance	Co. E, 26th NCT
9	Andrews, James T. (4)	Nash	Co. K, 12th NCT
10	Angel, D. W.	Orange	
11	Anthony, Abraham (4) (also Abram)	Catawba	Co. E, 32nd NCT
12	Anthony, Miller	Lincoln	Co. M, 16th NCT
13	Apple, William Mebane (2)	Guilford	Co. I, 8th NCST
14	Archer, Cyrus (2) (also Archie)	Mecklenburg	Co. H, 7th NCST
15	Archy, Josiah	Cabarrus	
16	Arney—see also Earney		

	Date	Limb	Location
1	3 June 1867 6 June 1867	Arm	CW Military 41 Aud. 6.1, p. 1
2	20 Feb 1866 9 April 1867	Arm	Worth 1, Co. List Aud. 6.1, p. 1
3	24 Feb 1866	Arm	Worth 1, Co. List
4	19 April 1866 25 March 1867 6 April 1867	Arm	CW Military 41 CW Mil, Co. List CW Military 41
5	12 March 1866 22 Aug 1866 25 Aug 1866 6 Oct 1866 9 Oct 1866 13 Oct 1866 17 March 1868 13 May 1868	Leg	CW Mil, Co. List Worth 3, form Worth 3, letter AG 58, p. 153 Aud. 6.1, p. 1 Jewett Invoices CW Military 41 CW Military 41
6	31 May 1866 1 May 1867	Arm	Worth 2, Co. List Aud. 6.1, p. 1
7	9 Nov 1866		Worth 4, Co. List
8	5 Jan. 1867	Leg	Aud. 6.1, p. 1
9	19 July 1866 23 July 1866 24 Aug 1866 (2)	Leg	Worth 3, form Worth 3, letter Jewett Invoices Aud. 6.1, p. 1
10	23 July 1867	Arm	CW Military 41
11	24 Feb 1866 8 June 1866 31 Oct 1866 (2)	Leg	Worth 1, Co. List Worth 3, order Jewett Invoices Aud. 6.1, p. 1
12	20 Aug 1867	Arm	Aud. 6.1, p. 1
13	7 March 1867 no date	Arm	Aud. 6.1, p. 1 Worth 8, Co. List
14	9 Nov 1866 18 April 1867	Arm	Worth 4, Co. List Aud. 6.1, p. 1
15	26 March 1866	Arm	Worth 2, Co. List
16			

	Claimant	County	Confederate Unit
1	Arney, George (4)	Caldwell	Co. F, 26th NCT
2	Arnt, John M. (5)	Catawba	Co. A, 12th NCT
3	Ashel, William	Randolph	
4	Atkins, Neill (3)	Harnett	Co. I, 15th NCT
5	Aubry, William (2) (also Aubery)	Surry	
6	Austin, John M.	Stanly	Co. I, 52nd NCT
7	Austin, Mark	Stanly	
8	Austin, Milton S.	Richmond	Co. E, 52nd NCT
9	Austin, Thomas A. (2)	Mitchell	Co. B, 15th NCT
10	Autry, W. W. (2)	Cumberland	Co. C, 54th NCT
11	Ayers, Hardy (5) (also Hardie)	Guilford	Co. B, 27th NCT
12	Badger, Sidney A. (4)	Caldwell	Co. F, 26th NCT
13	Baker, C. H.	Nash	Co. C, 1st NCST
14	Baker, George (3)	Halifax	Capt. Haskell's Lt. Arty.

	Date	Limb	Location
1	12 July 1866 4 Dec 1866 10 Jan 1867 (2)	Leg	Worth 3, form CW Military 41 Jewett Invoices Aud. 6.1, p. 1
2	24 Feb 1866 28 Sept 1866 8 Jan 1867 (2) 9 Nov 1868	Leg	Worth 1, Co. List Worth 3, form Jewett Invoices Aud. 6.1, p. 1 CW Military 41
3	29 Oct 1866	Wrist	Worth 3, Co. List
4	5 Feb 1866 28 Sept 1867 2 Oct 1867	Arm	Worth 1, Co. List CW Military 41 Aud. 6.1, p. 2
5	26 May 1866 1 June 1866	Leg	Worth 2, letter Aud. 6.1, p. 1
6	13 March 1867	Arm	Aud. 6.1, p. 2
7	24 Feb 1866	Arm	Worth 1, Co. List
8	25 March 1881	Arm	CW Military 41
9	5 April 1867 25 April 1867	Arm	CW Military 41 Aud. 6.1, p. 1
10	24 May 1866 26 Sept 1866	Leg	Worth 2, form Aud. 6.1, p. 1
11	16 Aug 1866 21 Aug 1866 15 Sept 1866 18 Dec 1867 no date	Leg	Worth 3, form CW Military 41 AG 58, p. 82 Aud. 6.1, p. 1 Worth 8, Co. List
12	7 July 1866 21 Nov 1866 8 Jan 1867 (2)	Leg	Worth 3, form CW Military 41 Jewett Invoices Aud. 6.1, p. 4
13	13 April 1867	Arm	Aud. 6.1, p. 6
14	5 March 1866 8 Oct 1870 13 Oct 1870	Arm	Worth 2, Co. List Aud. 6.1, p. 62 TC $ Bk 4, p. 449

	Claimant	County	Confederate Unit
1	Baker, H. C. (5)	Yadkin	Co. F, 28th NCT
2	Baker, John A. (8)	Franklin	Co. K, 24th NCT
3	Baker, Jonas (4) *(see also George Wright in CW Mil. 41)	Cleveland	Co. C, 38th NCT
4	Baker, Laurence S. [Col.]	Gates	9th NCST (1st NC Cav.)
5	Baker, R. J. (2)	Cumberland	Co. A, 51st NCT
6	Baldwin, Joseph R. (6) (The leg was returned in 1868 for $50 commutation.)	Ashe	Co. A, 26th NCT
7	Balkcum, William	Johnston	Co. F, 20th NCT
8	Ball, Daniel N. (3)	Iredell	Co. H, 4th NCST
9	Ball, Elijah Y. (3)	Iredell	Co. H, 44th NCT
10	Ball, Lemuel D. (2)	Granville	Co. I, 55th NCT
11	Ball, Robert (2)	Warren	[Co. E], 9th NCST (1st NC Cav.)

	Date	Limb	Location
1	Sept 1866 7 Sept 1866 6 Oct 1866 17 Oct 1866 (2)	Leg	AG 58, p. 120 Worth 3, letter AG 58, p. 161 Jewett Invoices Aud. 6.1, p. 3
2	2 Oct 1866 (2) 6 Oct 1866 (2) 13 Oct 1866 16 Oct 1866 25 Oct 1866 (2)	Leg	CW Military 41 AG 58, p. 163 AG 58, p. 164 AG 58, p. 175 CW Military 41 CW Military 41 Aud. 6.1, p. 4
3	13 Aug 1867 (2) 9 March 1868 no date	Hand	CW Military 41* Aud. 6.1, p. 7 CW Military 41 CW Military 41
4	7 April 1883	Arm	CW Military 41
5	28 July 1866 (2)	Leg	Jewett Invoices Aud. 6.1, p. 3
6	7 April 1866 16 June 1866 18 Dec 1866 (2) 16 Jan 1868 (2)	Leg	Worth 2, Co. List Worth 3, form Jewett Invoices Aud. 6.1, p. 3 Worth 8, letter Aud. 6.1, p. 62
7	8 June 1867	Arm	Aud. 6.1, p. 6
8	3 April 1866 1 March 1867 4 March 1867	Arm	Worth 2, Co. List CW Military 41 Aud. 6.1, p. 5
9	3 April 1866 1 March 1867 4 March 1867	Arm	Worth 2, Co. List CW Military 41 Aud. 6.1, p. 5
10	8 April 1867 6 May 1867	Arm	CW Military 41 Aud. 6.1, p. 6
11	25 March 1867 9 Sept 1867	Arm	Worth 4, letter Aud. 6.1, p. 7

	Claimant	County	Confederate Unit
1	Ballew, William J. (2)	Jackson	Co. A, 16th NCT
2	Bantey, N.	Northampton	
3	Barbee, Josiah	Stanly	Co. B, 5th NCST
4	Barber, Joseph	Rowan	Co. B, 4th NCST
5	Barefoot, Nathan	Sampson	Co. B, 56th NCT
6	Barham, Irwin H.	Halifax	
7	Barham, Junius H. (5)	Northampton	Co. H, 2nd NCST
8	Barham, W. L. (2)	Rockingham	Co. G, 45th NCT
9	Barham, William R.	Hertford	Co. F, 1st NCST
10	Barlow, William (3)	Wake	Co. E, 14th NCT
11	Barnes, J. M.	Stokes	Co. H, 23rd Va. Bat.
12	Barnett, James (3)	Duplin	Co. D, 27th NCT
13	Barnett, N. B. (3) (also N. P.)	Henderson	Co. I, 16th NCT
14	Barnhardt, A. B. (2) (also Barnhart)	Cabarrus	Co. H, 8th NCST
15	Barnhardt, Paul (2)	Cabarrus	Co. L, 17th NCT
16	Barrow, James E. (4)	Forsyth	Co. D, 57th NCT (He is also erroneously reported to have been in the 31st NCT.)
17	Bass, Henry	Surry	Co. B, 2nd Bn. NC Inf.

	Date	Limb	Location
1	4 June 1867 1 July 1867	Leg	CW Military 41 Aud. 6.1, p. 6
2	1 May 1866	Arm	Worth 2, Co. List
3	27 Aug 1867	Leg	Aud. 6.1, p. 7
4	19 March 1867	Arm	Aud. 6.1, p. 5
5	18 March 1867	Arm	Aud. 6.1, p. 5
6	27 Aug 1866	Leg	AG 58, p. 100
7	1 May 1866 30 July 1866 (2) 30 Aug 1866 (2)	Leg	Worth 2, Co. List Worth 3, form Jewett Invoices Aud. 6.1, p. 3
8	8 July 1867 (2)	Arm	CW Military 41 Aud. 6.1, p. 7
9	26 Dec 1866	Legs	Aud. 6.1, p. 3
10	19 March 1867 (2) no date		CW Military 41 Aud. 6.1, p. 5 CW Mil, Co. List
11	1 July 1867	Arm	Aud. 6.1, p. 6
12	19 April 1866 22 Feb 1867 (2)	Arm	CW Military 41, CW Mil, Co. List Aud. 6.1, p. 5
13	16 April 1866 2 March 1867 12 March 1867	Arm	Worth 2, Co. List CW Military 41 Aud. 6.1, p. 4
14	30 Jan 1867 31 Jan 1867	Leg	CW Military 41 Aud. 6.1, p. 3
15	26 March 1866 25 April 1867	Arm	Worth 2, Co. List Aud. 6.1, p. 6
16	8 March 1866 23 June 1866 25 Aug 1866 (2)	Leg	Worth 2, Co. List Worth 3, form Jewett Invoices Aud. 6.1, p. 3
17	29 Oct 1867	Arm	Aud. 6.1, p. 7

	Claimant	County	Confederate Unit
1	Bass, J. M.	Sampson	Co. C, 7th NCST
2	Batchelor, Henry	Nash	Co. I, 30th NCT
3	Batten, William W. (3)	Johnston	Co. C, 1st NCST
4	Baucom, Riley	Union	Co. C, 10th Bn. NC Heavy Arty.
5	Bean, W. H. (2)	Rowan	[Co. K], 8th NCST
6	Beatty, Andrew (2) (also Beattie)	Gaston	Co. B, 28th NCT
7	Beaver, James W. (3) (also Beavers)	Person	Co. A, 24th NCT
8	Beck, George L. (4)	Forsyth	Co. D, 57th NCT
9	Beck, William H. (4)	Davie	Co. G, 4th NCST
10	Beck, William T.	Davie	
11	Beeman, H. C. (5) (erroneously listed as H. C. Breeman on invoice)	Anson	Co. H, 43rd NCT
12	Belk, Darling	Union	[Co. F, 48th NCT]
13	Belk, Samuel E. (4) (also Belt)	Mecklenburg	Co. B, 53rd NCT
14	Bell, Eli (2)	Gaston	[Co. H, 21st NCT]

	Date	Limb	Location
1	30 July 1881	Hand	CW Military 41
2	13 April 1867	Arm	Aud. 6.1, p. 6
3	2 March 1867 11 March 1867 28 March 1867	Arm	CW Military 41 Worth 4, letter Aud. 6.1, p. 5
4	22 Feb 1867	Arm	Aud. 6.1, p. 4
5	23 April 1866 1 April 1867	Leg	CW Mil, Co. List Aud. 6.1, p. 4
6	6 April 1867 no date	Arm	Aud. 6.1, p. 4 Worth 8, Co. List
7	27 Nov 1866 22 July 1867 30 Aug 1867	Leg	Worth 4, Co. List CW Military 41 Aud. 6.1, p. 7
8	8 March 1866 13 April 1867 25 April 1867 3 May 1867	Arm	Worth 2, Co. List CW Military 41 Aud. 6.1, p. 6 CW Military 41
9	13 March 1866 30 June 1866 10 Oct 1866 (2)	Leg	Worth 2, Co. List Worth 3, form Jewett Invoices Aud. 6.1, p. 3
10	27 Aug 1866	Leg	AG 58, p. 102
11	9 June 1866 24 Aug 1866 Sept 1866 6 Nov 1866 (2)	Leg	Worth 3, form CW Military 41 AG 58, p. 109 Jewett Invoices Aud. 6.1, p. 4
12	22 Oct 1866	Leg	Worth 3, Co. List
13	9 Nov 1866 19 March 1867 22 March 1867 2 April 1867	Arm	Worth 4, Co. List CW Military 41 Aud. 6.1, p. 7 CW Military 41
14	1 March 1867 (2)	Arm	CW Military 41 Aud. 6.1, p. 5

	Claimant	County	Confederate Unit
1	Bell, L. M. (4)	Chester, S.C., and Gaston	Co. B, 28th NCT
2	Bell, Thomas S.	Wilkes	Co. B, 55th NCT
3	Bell, Walter R. (5)	Duplin	Co. B, 51st NCT
4	Belo, R. W. (3)	Forsyth	Co. H, 56th NCT
5	Belvin, T. H.	Wake	Co. I, 3rd NCST
6	Belvings, Calvin	Ashe	Co. A, 26th NCT
7	Bennett, D. K.	Brunswick	
8	Bennett, Frank (2)	Anson	[Co. A, 23rd NCT]
9	Bennett, Joseph J.	Wake	Co. A, 4th NCST
10	Benton, Seabron A. (3) (also Seaborn)	Anson	Co. K, 26th NCT
11	Berrier, Hiram R. (3)	Davidson	Co. B, 10th Va. Cav.
12	Best, A. J.	Gaston	Co. B, 28th NCT
13	Best, T. W. (3)	Wayne	Co. F, 7th NCST
14	Bethune, David (6)	Robeson	Co. G, 24th NCT

	Date	Limb	Location
1	20 Feb 1867 27 Feb 1867 9 March 1867 no date	Arm	CW Military 41 Aud. 6.1, p. 5 Worth 4, letter Worth 8, Co. List
2	6 Nov 1867	Hand	Aud. 6.1, p. 7
3	19 April 1866 4 March 1867 14 March 1867 20 March 1867 6 April 1867	Arm	CW Military 41 CW Mil, Co. List Aud. 6.1, p. 5 CW Military 41 CW Military 41
4	8 March 1866 25 June 1866 29 Sept 1866	Leg	Worth 2, Co. List Worth 3, form Aud. 6.1, p. 4
5	22 May 1867	Arm	Aud. 6.1, p. 6
6	16 July 1866	Leg	Aud. 6.1, p. 3
7	22 Feb 1868	Arm	CW Military 41
8	30 March 1867 5 April 1867	Arm	CW Military 41 Aud. 6.1, p. 4
9	2 April 1867	Arm	Aud. 6.1, p. 4
10	16 June 1866 9 Jan 1867 (2)	Leg	Worth 3, form Jewett Invoices Aud. 6.1, p. 3
11	21 May 1866 22 Dec 1866 (2)	Leg	Worth 2, letter Jewett Invoices Aud. 6.1, p. 4
12	27 Feb 1867	Arm	Aud. 6.1, p. 5
13	2 Nov 1867 7 Nov 1867 (2)	Arm	CW Military 41 Aud. 6.1, p. 7 CW Military 41
14	21 Feb 1866 3 July 1866 18 Aug 1866 10 Oct 1866 30 Oct 1866 (2)	Leg	Worth 1, Co. List Worth 3, form Worth 3, letter Worth 3, Co. List Jewett Invoices Aud. 6.1, p. 3

	Claimant	County	Confederate Unit
1	Bevil, John (2) (also J. L. C. Berrill)	Rockingham	Co. E, 45th NCT
2	Bickett, Nimrod J.	Union	Co. A, 48th NCT
3	Biggerstaff, G. M.	Rutherford	Co. C, 15th NCT
4	Billingsby, James M. (2)	Anson	[Co. A, 23rd NCT]
5	Bishop, James H. (4)	Duplin	Co. C, 66th NCT
6	Bivens, Joseph A. (3)	Union	Co. I, 53rd NCT
7	Black, John (3)	Ashe	Co. A, 37th NCT
8	Black, John	Rowan	Co. C, 42nd NCT
9	Blalock, John B. (2)	Cleveland	Co. B, 28th NCT
10	Blalock, M. V.	Orange	Co. C, 6th NCST
11	Bland, C. C. (3)	Pitt	Co. K, [36th NCT (2nd NC Arty.)]
12	Blankenship, Robert B. (4)	Yancey	
13	Blevins, Calvin (3) (also Bleving)	Ashe	Co. A, 26th NCT
14	Blevins, Felix (2) * (Cash book indicates payment for an *arm*. It was likely a $50 commutation. All other sources list foot.)	Ashe	[Co. A, 26th NCT]

	Date	Limb	Location
1	12 March 1866 20 April 1867	Arm	CW Mil, Co. List Aud. 6.1, p. 6
2	8 Aug 1866	Leg	Aud. 6.1, p. 3
3	7 May 1867	Arm	Aud. 6.1, p. 7
4	23 March 1867 27 March 1867	Arm	CW Military 41 Aud. 6.1, p. 4
5	19 April 1866 15 July 1867 (2) 28 Nov 1867	Leg	CW Mil, Co. List Jewett Invoices Aud. 6.1, p. 3 CW Military 41
6	22 Oct 1866 21 Feb 1867 (2)	Arm	Worth 3, Co. List Aud. 6.1, p. 4 CW Mil, Co. List
7	7 April 1866 25 Sept 1867 2 Oct 1867	Leg	Worth 2, Co. List CW Military 41 Aud. 6.1, p. 7
8	19 March 1867	Arm	Aud. 6.1, p. 5
9	8 April 1867 no date	Arm	Aud. 6.1, p. 5 Worth 8, Co. List
10	19 April 1867	Leg	Aud. 6.1, p. 6
11	24 Aug 1866 3 Nov 1866 5 Nov 1866	Leg	AG 58, p. 88 Aud. 6.1, p. 3 Jewett Invoices
12	5 June 1867 8 Nov 1867 23 Nov 1867 14 March 1868	Leg	CW Military 41 Worth 7, letter Aud. 6.1, p. 7 CW Military 41
13	7 April 1866 16 July 1866 10 Dec 1868	Leg	Worth 2, Co. List Jewett Invoices CW Military 41
14	14 Nov 1866 5 Jan 1869	Foot*	CW Military 41 TC $ Bk 4, p. 181

	Claimant	County	Confederate Unit
1	Blinson, James M. (2)	Wake	Co. D, 31st NCT
2	Boger, G. C. (3) (erroneously listed as Boyer on invoice)	Iredell	Co. H, 2nd NCST
3	Boggs, Peter F. (4)	Ashe	[Co. A, 9th NCST (1st NC Cav.)]
4	Bolejack, W. E. (4) (also Boleyjack)	Forsyth	Co. G, 21st NCT
5	Bolick, J. A.	Caldwell	Co. H, 58th NCT
6	Boling, Nicholas (3)	Chatham	Co. H, 47th NCT
7	Boon, Henry	Nash	Co. E, 7th NCST
8	Boon, W. Joseph (4)	Chatham	Co. A, 5th NCST
9	Bost, Harvey	Catawba	[Co. A, 12th NCT]
10	Bost, Henry M. (6)	Cabarrus	Co. F, 9th NCST (1st NC Cav.)
11	Bost, J. H. (2)	Catawba	Co. A, 12th NCT
12	Bostick, Bryant W. (4) (also Bryan Bostick)	Duplin	Co. E, 30th NCT
13	Bowen, Richard (3)	Person	Co. A, 24th NCT

	Date	Limb	Location
1	20 March 1867 (2)	Arm	CW Military 41 Aud. 6.1, p. 5
2	3 April 1866 20 Nov 1866 (2)	Leg	Worth 2, Co. List Jewett Invoices Aud. 6.1, p. 4
3	7 April 1866 26 March 1867 1 April 1867 6 April 1867	Leg	Worth 2, Co. List CW Military 41 Aud. 6.1, p. 4 CW Military 41
4	8 March 1866 27 June 1866 26 July 1866 (2)	Foot	Worth 2, Co. List Worth 3, form Jewett Invoices Aud. 6.1, p. 3
5	26 April 1867	Arm	Aud. 6.1, p. 6
6	17 June 1868 (3)	Leg	Worth 8, letter TC $ Bk 4, p. 93 Aud. 6.1, p. 62
7	1 Jan 1868	Leg	Aud. 6.1, p. 7
8	5 Dec 1866 14 Feb 1867 25 May 1867 (2)	Leg	Worth 4, Co. List CW Military 41 Jewett Invoices Aud. 6.1, p. 4
9	24 Feb 1866	Arm	Worth 1, Co. List
10	26 March 1866 15 Nov 1866 16 Nov 1866 28 Nov 1866 (2) 24 April 1867	Leg	Worth 2, Co. List CW Military 41 Worth 4, letter Jewett Invoices Aud. 6.1, p. 4 CW Military 41
11	1 May 1867 4 May 1867	Arm	CW Military 41 Aud. 6.1, p. 6
12	19 April 1866 8 April 1867 11 April 1867 20 April 1867		CW Mil, Co. List Worth 5, letter Aud. 6.1, p. 4 CW Military 41
13	27 Nov 1866 2 April 1867 (2)	Arm	Worth 4, Co. List CW Military 41 Aud. 6.1, p. 5

	Claimant	County	Confederate Unit
1	Boyet, John M.	Anson	Co. K, 26th NCT
2	Bradley, John H. (4)	Rutherford	Co. G, 16th NCT
3	Bradshaw, David W. (2)	Duplin	Co. A, 43rd NCT
4	Brady, B. B.	Randolph	Co. L, 22nd NCT
5	Bragg, Thomas W. (2)	Granville	Co. I, 55th NCT
6	Branowski, John N. (7) (also Branoski)	Halifax and Warren	Co. G, 61st Va.
7	Brantley, Alexander	Rowan	
8	Brantley, S. G. (2)	Rowan	Co. C, 33rd NCT
9	Brewer, Thomas (3)	Northampton	[Co. E, 56th NCT]
10	Brewer, William T. (2)	Hertford	
11	Brewer, William Thomas	Northampton	Co. A, 56th NCT
12	Bridges, H. H.	Cleveland	Co. G, 18th NCT
13	Bridges, John M. (4)	Cleveland	Co. I, 38th NCT (erroneously reported as 30th NCT in Aud.)
14	Bridges, T. W.	Cleveland	Co. H, 28th NCT
15	Brinkley, Henry B. (3)	Davidson	Co. B, 48th NCT

	Date	Limb	Location
1	29 March 1867	Arm	Aud. 6.1, p. 4
2	26 June 1866 8 Aug 1866 16 Oct 1866 (2)	Leg	Worth 3, order AG 58, p. 55 Jewett Invoices Aud. 6.1, p. 3
3	10 July 1867 (2)	Arm	CW Military 41 Aud. 6.1, p. 6
4	3 April 1868	Arm	Aud. 6.1, p. 7
5	12 March 1866 8 April 1867	Arm	Worth 2, Co. List Aud. 6.1, p. 5
6	5 March 1866 15 May 1866 26 June 1866 [Sept 1866] 25 Sept 1866 (2) 31 July 1867	Leg	Worth 2, Co. List CW Military 41 Worth 3, form AG 58, p. 135 Jewett Invoices Aud. 6.1, p. 3
7	23 April 1866	Leg	CW Mil, Co. List
8	3 July 1866 (2)	Leg	Jewett Invoices Aud. 6.1, p. 4
9	1 May 1866 27 Sept 1867 (2)	Arm	Worth 2, Co. List CW Military 41 Aud. 6.1, p. 7
10	26 Dec 1866 26 Feb 1867	Arm	CW Military 41 Aud. 6.1, p. 5
11	29 Oct 1867	Arm	CW Military 41
12	6 April 1867	Arm	Aud. 6.1, p. 5
13	23 Nov 1866 11 Dec 1866 (2) no date	Leg	CW Military 41 Jewett Invoices Aud. 6.1, p. 3 Worth 8, Co. List
14	27 Feb 1867	Arm	Aud. 6.1, p. 5
15	2 March 1867 4 May 1867 (2)	Arm	CW Military 41 Jewett Invoices Aud. 6.1, p. 5

	Claimant	County	Confederate Unit
1	Brinson, James	Wake	
2	Broadhurst, David J. (2)	Duplin	Co. K, 20th NCT
3	Brock, Robert	Wayne	Co. C, 28th NCT
4	Brookfield, Rayner (2)	Craven	Co. F, 20th NCT
5	Brooks, William F., Capt.	Brunswick	Co. K, 36th NCT
6	Brookshire, F. W. (2)	Alexander	Co. D, 18th NCT
7	Broom, A. T. (6) (erroneously listed as A. T. Brown in Aud.)	Union	Co. B, 43rd NCT
8	Broom, Philip	Buncombe	Co. A, 48th NCT
9	Brown, Abner L.	Cabarrus	Co. A, 2nd NCST
10	Brown, Evan	Orange	Co. G, 27th NCT
11	Brown, H. C. (2)	Guilford	Co. C, 45th NCT
12	Brown, Isaac (6) *(see also Walter R. Bell in CW Military 41)	Duplin	Co. A, 43rd NCT
13	Brown, Isaac H. (2)	New Hanover	Co. K, 3rd NCST
14	Brown, J. S. (2)	Cabarrus	Co. A, 24th NCT
15	Brown, James J. (3)	Mecklenburg	Co. D, 7th NCST

	Date	Limb	Location
1	no date	Arm	CW Mil, Co. List
2	9 April 1867 11 April 1867	Arm	CW Military 41 Aud. 6.1, p. 6
3	30 April 1867	Arm	Aud. 6.1, p. 6
4	21 Aug 1866 19 Oct 1866	Leg	Worth 3, form Aud. 6.1, p. 3
5	3 June 1868	Arm	CW Military 41
6	11 Nov 1867 (2)	Hand	CW Military 41 Aud. 6.1, p. 60
7	6 June 1866 20 Aug 1866 27 Aug 1866 6 Oct 1866 10 Oct 1866 (2)	Leg	Worth 3, form Worth 3, letter AG 58, p. 92 AG 58, p. 159 Jewett Invoices Aud. 6.1, p. 3
8	1 May 1867	Arm	Aud. 6.1, p. 6
9	6 April 1867	Arm	Aud. 6.1, p. 4
10	27 March 1867	Arm	Aud. 6.1, p. 5
11	no date 14 March 1867	Arm	Worth 8, City List Aud. 6.1, p. 5
12	19 April 1866 18 March 1867 22 March 1867 30 March 1867 8 April 1867 10 April 1869	Arm	CW Military 41* CW Mil, Co. List Aud. 6.1, p. 5 CW Military 41 CW Military 41 CW Military 41
13	20 March 1867 1 April 1867	Arm	CW Military 41 Aud. 6.1, p. 4
14	30 March 1868 31 March 1868	Arm	CW Military 41 Aud. 6.1, p. 7
15	9 Nov 1866 23 Jan 1868 (2)	Leg	Worth 4, Co. List Worth 8, letter Aud. 6.1, p. 7

	Claimant	County	Confederate Unit
1	Brown, James T. (2) *(see also Ira T. Hardison in CW Military 41)	Martin	17th NCT
2	Brown, Simon (4)	Johnston	Co. C, 53rd NCT
3	Brown, Stanhope	Mecklenburg	Co. H, 35th NCT
4	Brown, Stephen W. (2)	Richmond	Co. F, 18th NCT
5	Brown, William	Edgecombe	Co. B, 44th NCT
6	Brown, William H. (2)	Hertford	Co. D, 59th NCT (4th NC Cav.)
7	Brown, William S.	Mecklenburg	Co. K, 56th NCT
8	Bryan, David (3) (also Bryant)	Bladen	[2nd] Co. I, 36th NCT
9	Bryan, Gaston (2) (also Gladson Byron)	Rockingham	Co. A, 66th NCT
10	Bryant, Augustus (3)	Wilson	Co. B, 47th NCT
11	Buck, Bryan (5)	Beaufort	Co. E, 59th NCT (4th NC Cav.)
12	Buff, David (2)	Cleveland	Co. F, 55th NCT
13	Bullard, Alvin (5) *(see also Jordan Powers in CW Military 41)	Columbus	[Co. K, 20th NCT, listed as Alva]
14	Bullock, Jesse B.	Pitt	Co. E, 3rd NCST

	Date	Limb	Location
1	24 Aug 1867 27 Sept 1867	Arm	CW Military 41* Aud. 6.1, p. 7
2	5 March 1866 8 Aug 1866 18 Aug 1866 no date	Leg	Worth 2, Co. List AG 58, p. 57 Jewett Invoices Aud. 6.1, p. 7
3	12 Dec 1867	Arm	Aud. 6.1, p. 7
4	15 April 1867 25 April 1867	Legs	CW Military 41 Aud. 6.1, p. 6
5	10 Oct 1867	Hand	CW Military 41
6	28 Feb 1868 29 Feb 1868	Arm	CW Military 41 Aud. 6.1, p. 7
7	10 April 1867	Arm	Aud. 6.1, p. 5
8	10 April 1866 6 May 1867 8 May 1867	Arm	Worth 2, Co. List CW Military 41 Aud. 6.1, p. 6
9	8 July 1867 (2)	Arm	CW Military 41 Aud. 6.1, p. 6
10	13 Dec 1866 7 Jan 1867 (2)	Leg	CW Military 41 Jewett Invoices Aud. 6.1, p. 3
11	6 April 1867 12 April 1867 15 April 1867 20 May 1867 28 May 1867	Hand	CW Military 41 Aud. 6.1, p. 6 CW Military 41 CW Military 41 CW Military 41
12	21 Sept 1867 22 Sept 1867	Arm	CW Military 41 Aud. 6.1, p. 7
13	8 April 1867 25 April 1867 26 April 1867 19 July 1867 no date	Leg	Worth 5, form CW Military 41* Aud. 6.1, p. 6 CW Military 41 CW Military 41
14	19 March 1867	Arm	Aud. 6.1, p. 4

	Claimant	County	Confederate Unit
1	Burgin, S. W. (3)	Buncombe	Co. F, 3rd Ala.
2	Burke, Henry F. (4)	Forsyth	Co. K, 48th NCT
3	Burkett, David	Davidson	Co. I, 42nd NCT
4	Burkhart, Edward F. (3)	Davidson	Co. H, 48th NCT
5	Burkhart, James F.	Davidson	Co. I, 42nd NCT
6	Burns, Elisha (2)	Chatham	Co. G, 48th NCT
7	Busick, D. W. (4) (Danl. on Co. List; Durant W. in *NCT Roster*)	Guilford	Co. E, 22nd NCT (erroneously reported as Co. E, 33rd NCT, in Aud.)
8	Busick, William H.	Guilford	
9	Butcher, James (2)	Surry	Co. A, 28th NCT
10	Butler, Irvin (2) (also Irwin)	Burke	Co. D, 11th NCT
11	Butler, John R. (2)	Rutherford	Co. D, 16th NCT
12	Bynum, J. R.	Warren	Co. C, 12th NCT
13	Byrd, George J. (3)	Cumberland	[Co. E], 56th NCT [Co. E, 10th NCST (1st NC Arty.)]
14	Byrd, James H. (3) (also Bird)	McDowell	Co. A, 49th NCT

	Date	Limb	Location
1	10 May 1866 8 Dec 1866 (2)	Leg	Worth 2, Co. List Jewett Invoices Aud. 6.1, p. 3
2	8 March 1866 14 June 1866 21 Aug 1866 (2)	Leg	Worth 2, Co. List Worth 3, form Jewett Invoices Aud. 6.1, p. 3
3	19 Sept 1868	Arm	Aud. 6.1, p. 62
4	1 July 1868 (3)	Arm	CW Military 41 TC $ Bk 4, p. 97 Aud. 6.1, p. 62
5	21 Feb 1867	Arm	Aud. 6.1, p. 4
6	13 July 1867 13 Aug 1867	Leg	CW Military 41 Aud. 6.1, p. 6
7	18 Oct 1866 (2) no date (2)	Leg	Jewett Invoices Aud. 6.1, p. 3 Worth 8, Co. List and City List
8	no date	Leg	Worth 8, City List
9	23 Feb 1867 (2)	Arm	CW Military 41 Aud. 6.1, p. 7
10	23 July 1867 (2)	Arm	CW Military 41 Aud. 6.1, p. 6
11	22 Aug 1867 (2)	Left foot	CW Military 41 Aud. 6.1, p. 7
12	1 June 1867	Arm	Aud. 6.1, p. 6
13	11 June 1866 4 Aug 1866 (2)	Leg	Worth 3, order Jewett Invoices Aud. 6.1, p. 4
14	31 May 1866 8 Jan 1867 (2)	Leg	Worth 2, Co. List Jewett Invoices Aud. 6.1, p. 3

	Claimant	County	Confederate Unit
1	Byrd, Robert (3)	McDowell	[Co. D], 25th NCT
2	Byrns, Mat. (2)	Columbus	Co. H, 18th NCT
3	Caddell, George K. (3) (erroneously listed as Caldwell in Aud.)	Anson	Co. K, 43rd NCT
4	Cahill, Timothy J. (5)	Mecklenburg	Co. D, 7th NCST
5	Cain, Anderson (5) (also N. A. Cain) (1869 paymt. was likely for the return of the leg.)	Orange and Wilkes	Co. F, 52nd NCT
6	Calaway, James	Alleghany	Co. D, 61st NCT
7	Calaway, James	Person	Co. D, 61st NCT
8	Caldwell, A. B.	Mecklenburg	
9	Caldwell, John	Alleghany	Co. I, 37th NCT
10	Caldwell, M. B. (3)	Mecklenburg	Co. K, 23rd NCT
11	Callaway, James W. (5)	Alleghany	Co. D, 11th NCT
12	Calloway, J. W. (3)	Madison	Co. B, 16th NCT
13	Camp, Henry A.	Rowan	Co. G, 18th Ark.

	Date	Limb	Location
1	2 May 1868 30 May 1868 (2)	Arm	CW Military 41 TC $ Bk 4, p. 89 Aud. 6.1, p. 62
2	21 Feb 1867 26 Feb 1867	Arm	CW Military 41 Aud. 6.1, p. 5
3	8 June 1866 8 Jan 1867 (2)	Leg	Worth 3, form Jewett Invoices Aud. 6.1, p. 9
4	18 June 1866 24 Aug 1866 9 Nov 1866 5 Dec 1866 (2)	Leg	Worth 3, form AG 58, p. 95 Worth 4, Co. List Jewett Invoices Aud. 6.1, p. 8
5	30 Aug 1866 (2) 1 Nov 1866 27 July 1867 2 Aug. 1869	Leg	Jewett Invoices Aud. 6.1, p. 8 Worth 4, Co. List Worth 6, letter TC $ Bk 4, p. 269
6	21 Sept 1867	Arm	CW Military 41
7	27 Sept 1867	Arm	Aud. 6.1, p. 11
8	9 Nov 1866	Leg	Worth 4, Co. List
9	28 Feb 1867	Leg	Aud. 6.1, p. 12
10	19 July 1866 3 Dec 1866 (2)	Leg	Worth 3, form Jewett Invoices Aud. 6.1, p. 8
11	25 Nov 1867 17 Feb 1868 16 March 1868 1 May 1868 11 June 1868	Arm	CW Military 41 TC $ Bk 4, p. 93 Aud. 6.1, p. 12 CW Military 41 CW Military 41
12	29 Aug 1866 20 Dec 1866 (2)	Leg	AG 58, p. 104 Jewett Invoices Aud. 6.1, p. 8
13	25 June 1867	Leg	Aud. 6.1, p. 11

	Claimant	County	Confederate Unit
1	Camp, John (2)	Cleveland	Co. B, 26th NCT
2	Camp, Terrell (2)	Cleveland	Co. H, 34th NCT
3	Campbell, Enos L. (4)	Catawba and Lincoln	Co. E, 57th NCT
4	Campbell, John A.	Moore	Co. E, 11th NCT
5	Campbell, John Wesley (4)	Catawba	Co. E, 20th NCT
6	Campbell, W. R.	Chatham	Co. I, 32nd NCT
7	Campbell, William A.	Rowan	Co. D, 10th NCST (1st NC Arty.)
8	Canady, James (3)	Onslow	Co. B, 24th NCT
9	Canipe, David (2)	Lincoln	Co. F, 55th NCT
10	Cantrell, John	Rockingham	Co. E, 45th NCT
11	Canup, Henry A. (2)	Rowan	Co. G, 18th Ark.
12	Carroll, James H.	Warren	Co. F, 8th NCST
13	Carroll, Smith F. (3) (also Smith J.)	Watauga	
14	Carroll, Wiley	Wake	Co. E, 14th NCT
15	Carson, John B. (2)	Gaston	Co. B, 28th NCT
16	Carter, Isaac M.	Ashe	Co. A, 26th NCT
17	Carter, John E. (2)	Rowan	Co. D, 10th NCST (1st NC Arty.)

	Date	Limb	Location
1	12 March 1867 16 March 1867	Leg	CW Military 41 Aud. 6.1, p. 10
2	12 March 1867 16 March 1867	Arm	CW Military 41 Aud. 6.1, p. 10
3	24 Feb 1866 20 April 1867 25 April 1867 11 May 1867	Arm	Worth 1, Co. List CW Military 41 Aud. 6.1, p. 10 CW Military 41
4	31 May 1867	Arm	Aud. 6.1, p. 11
5	24 Feb 1866 13 April 1867 25 April 1867 1 May 1867	Arm	Worth 1, Co. List CW Military 41 CW Mil, Co. List Aud. 6.1, p. 10
6	21 June 1867	Leg	Aud. 6.1, p. 11
7	25 April 1867	Arm	Aud. 6.1, p. 10
8	3 Dec 1866 31 Jan 1867 (2)	Leg	CW Military 41 Jewett Invoices Aud. 6.1, p. 9
9	15 April 1867 4 May 1867	Arm	CW Military 41 Aud. 6.1, p. 11
10	20 May 1867	Arm	Aud. 6.1, p. 11
11	8 June 1867 10 June 1867	Leg	CW Military 41
12	2 Sept 1867	Arm	Aud. 6.1, p. 11
13	3 Oct 1866 6 Oct 1866 (2)	Leg	Worth 3, form CW Military 41 Aud. 6.1, p. 8
14	4 March 1867	Eyes	Aud. 6.1, p. 9
15	no date 27 Feb 1867	Arm	Worth 8, Co. List Aud. 6.1, p. 9
16	27 Dec 1866	Leg	Aud. 6.1, p. 9
17	23 April 1866 19 March 1867	Arm	CW Mil, Co. List Aud. 6.1, p. 8

	Claimant	County	Confederate Unit
1	Carter, John M.	Gaston	
2	Carter, Pleasant H.	Stokes	Co. H, 13th NCT
3	Carter, R. F. (2)	Cabarrus	Co. B, 20th NCT
4	Carter, S. S.	Alamance	Co. F, 66th NCT
5	Carter, William T. (4)	Rockingham	Co. G, 45th NCT
6	Carver, A. R., Capt. (2)	Cumberland	Co. B, 56th NCT
7	Carver, Dennis (3)	Person	[Co. E, 15th NCT]
8	Carver, Samuel (5)	Rockingham	Co. G, 45th NCT
9	Case, J. R.	Buncombe	
10	Case, Thomas D.	Buncombe	Co. D, 39th NCT
11	Cashion, J. H. (3)	Lincoln	Co. K, 63rd NCT (5th NC Cav.)
12	Cassel, Wesley (2)	Cabarrus	Co. H, 57th NCT
13	Cathey, Alexander A. (5)	Mecklenburg	Co. G, 34th NCT
14	Cathey, J. L. (4)	Buncombe	Co. I, 60th NCT

	Date	Limb	Location
1	8 Aug 1866	Leg	AG 58, p. 60
2	15 May 1867	Arm	Aud. 6.1, p. 11
3	26 July 1867 25 Aug 1867	Leg	CW Military 41 Aud. 6.1, p. 11
4	12 March 1867	Arm	Aud. 6.1, p. 10
5	12 March 1866 6 Aug 1866 31 Oct 1866 (2)	Leg	CW Mil, Co. List Worth 3, form Jewett Invoices Aud. 6.1, p. 8
6	3 July 1867 15 Aug 1867	Arm	Worth 6, letter Aud. 6.1, p. 11
7	27 Nov 1866 4 June 1867 (2)	Arm	Worth 4, Co. List CW Military 41 Aud. 6.1, p. 11
8	12 March 1866 8 Aug 1866 5 Oct 1866 16 Oct 1866 (2)	Leg	CW Mil, Co. List Worth 3, form AG 58, p. 148 Jewett Invoices Aud. 6.1, p. 8
9	10 May 1866	Arm	Worth 2, Co. List
10	3 April 1867	Leg	Aud. 6.1, p. 12
11	15 Nov 1866 (2) 6 May 1867	Leg	Jewett Invoices Aud. 6.1, p. 8 CW Military 41
12	26 March 1866 25 April 1867	Arm	Worth 2, Co. List Aud. 6.1, p. 10
13	5 June 1866 6 Oct 1866 30 Oct 1866 (2) 9 Nov 1866	Leg	Worth 3, form AG 58, p. 160 Jewett Invoices Aud. 6.1, p. 8 Worth 4, Co. List
14	10 May 1866 1 Jan 1867 (2) 22 Feb 1867	Leg	Worth 2, Co. List Jewett Invoices Aud. 6.1, p. 9 CW Military 41

	Claimant	County	Confederate Unit
1	Cathey, William (2)	Mecklenburg	Co. E, 19th NCT
2	Catlett, B. G.	Granville	Co. I, 55th NCT
3	Caudle, David (3) (also Cardel)	Chatham	Co. D, 61st NCT
4	Chamblee, B. D. (2)	Wake	Co. C, 24th NCT
5	Chamblee, W. B. (2) (also W. R.)	Wake	Co. B, 47th NCT
6	Chance, John R. (2)	Wayne	Co. G, 55th NCT
7	Chapel, Parks (3)	Richmond	[Co. D, 23rd NCT]
8	Chapman, Henry (4)	Union	Co. A, 48th NCT
9	Chappel, S. E. (2)	Wilkes	Co. G, 13th NCT
10	Cheely, A. C. (3)	Colorado Terr. (Guilford)	Co. B, 27th NCT
11	Cherry, Charles C. (4)	Edgecombe	Co. F, 36th NCT (2nd NC Arty.)
12	Cherry, M. L.	Pitt	Co. E, 55th NCT
13	Chilcutt, Franklin G. (3)	Guilford	Co. B, 27th NCT
14	Childers, B. F. (2)	Alexander	Co. K, 7th NCT

	Date	Limb	Location
1	9 Nov 1866 26 March 1867	Arm	Worth 4, Co. List Aud. 6.1, p. 10
2	8 April 1867	Arm	Aud. 6.1, p. 10
3	21 Sept 1866 (2) 5 Dec 1866	Leg	Jewett Invoices Aud. 6.1, p. 8 Worth 4, Co. List
4	8 June 1867 10 June 1867	Foot	CW Military 41 Aud. 6.1, p. 11
5	19 May 1867 20 May 1867	Leg	Aud. 6.1, p. 11 Worth 5, letter
6	19 April 1867 22 April 1867	Leg	CW Military 41 Aud. 6.1, p. 10
7	11 April 1866 23 Feb 1867 25 Feb 1867	Arm	Worth 2, Co. List Aud. 6.1, p. 9 CW Military 41
8	22 Oct 1866 25 March 1867 2 April 1867 15 April 1867	Arm	Worth 3, Co. List CW Military 41 Aud. 6.1, p. 10 CW Military 41
9	10 Oct 1867 (2)	Hand	CW Military 41 Aud. 6.1, p. 11
10	28 March 1867 no date (2)	Arm	CW Military 41 Worth 8, Co. List and City List
11	23 Sept 1866 27 Sept 1866 29 Oct 1866 (2)	Leg	CW Military 41 AG 58, p. 144 Jewett Invoices Aud. 6.1, p. 8
12	30 Oct 1866	Leg	Aud. 6.1, p. 8
13	no date 26 April 1867 (2)	Arm	Worth 8, Co. List Jewett Invoices Aud. 6.1, p. 10
14	25 Sept 1867 (2)	Hand	CW Military 41 Aud. 6.1, p. 11

	Claimant	County	Confederate Unit
1	Childers, N. A. (2)	Alexander	[Co. G], 37th NCT
2	Chisenhall, James R.	Orange	Co. D, 1st NC Inf. (6 months, 1861)
3	Christenbury, Samuel B. (3) (also Chrisenbury)	Mecklenburg	Co. C, 37th NCT
4	Clark, John O.	Orange	Co. D, 1st NCST
5	Clark, Richard F. (3)	Cleveland	Co. B, 49th NCT
6	Clark, Samuel (4)	Granville	Co. E, 23rd NCT
7	Clarke, S. M. (3)	Caldwell	Co. A, 22nd NCT
8	Clayton, Marion T. (5)	Person	Co. E, 35th NCT
9	Clements, William G. (2) (also Clemons)	Wake	Co. I, 6th NCST
10	Clifton, ————	Wake	
11	Clifton, Charles H.	Franklin	Co. F, 47th NCT
12	Clifton, Y. B. (2)	Wake	Co. I, 1st NCST
13	Clinton, Thadius L. (4)	Gaston	Co. H, 23rd NCT
14	Cloninger, Carry	Catawba	

	Date	Limb	Location
1	13 Feb 1867 23 Feb 1867	Leg	CW Military 41 Aud. 6.1, p. 9
2	12 Sept 1867		CW Military 41
3	9 Nov 1866 27 March 1867 1 April 1867	Arm	Worth 4, Co. List CW Military 41 Aud. 6.1, p. 10
4	27 March 1867	Arm	Aud. 6.1, p. 10
5	no date 23 May 1867 24 May 1867	Leg	Worth 8, Co. List CW Military 41 Aud. 6.1, p. 11
6	12 March 1866 14 June 1866 25 July 1866 (2)	Leg	Worth 2, Co. List Worth 3, form Jewett Invoices Aud. 6.1, p. 8
7	23 March 1867 5 June 1867 7 June 1867	Arm	CW Military 41 Aud. 6.1, p. 11 CW Military 41
8	19 June 1866 18 Oct 1866 29 Oct 1866 (2) 27 Nov 1866	Leg	Worth 3, form AG 58, p. 181 Jewett Invoices Aud. 6.1, p. 8 Worth 4, Co. List
9	5 April 1867 no date	Arm	Aud. 6.1, p. 10 CW Mil, Co. List
10	no date	Leg	CW Mil, Co. List
11	1 June 1867	Arm	Aud. 6.1, p. 11
12	6 June 1866 (2)	Leg	Jewett Invoices Aud. 6.1, p. 8
13	no date 24 Aug 1866 14 Sept 1866 (2)	Leg	Worth 8, Co. List AG 58, p. 89 Jewett Invoices Aud. 6.1, p. 8
14	24 Feb 1866	Arm	Worth 1, Co. List

	Claimant	County	Confederate Unit
1	Cloninger, Elkanah (2)	Catawba	Co. A, 12th NCT
2	Cobb, Henry L. (2)	Caswell	Co. D, 14th Tenn.
3	Cobb, John P. , Col.	Wayne	2nd NCST
4	Cobb, Kinchan (2)	Greene	Militia-see 1885 pension
5	Cobb, Stephan J. (Co. List indicates hand "disabled.")	Robeson	[Co. D, 51st NCT]
6	Coffey, B. M. (4)	Mecklenburg	Co. H, 17th NCT
7	Coffey, Rufus	Caldwell	Co. I, 26th NCT
8	Cole, Jesse W. (3)	Orange	Co. G, 28th NCT
9	Coleman, Josiah	Wilson	Co. B, 2nd NCST
10	Collins, James A. (3)	Alleghany	Co. A, 26th NCT
11	Collins, John (3)	Onslow	Co. B, 24th NCT
12	Collins, T. L. (2)	Halifax	
13	Collins, Thomas	Halifax	
14	Colville, James H. (2)	Harnett	Co. F, 15th NCT
15	Connor, H. W. (2)	Orange	Co. K, 23rd NCT
16	Conoly, Frank (Co. List indicates leg was "disabled.")	Robeson	[Co. D, 51st NCT]

	Date	Limb	Location
1	22 March 1867 2 April 1867	Arm	CW Military 41 Aud. 6.1, p. 10
2	20 Feb 1866 10 May 1867	Arm	Worth 1, Co. List Aud. 6.1, p. 10
3	16 Jan 1867	Leg	Aud. 6.1, p. 9
4	21 Feb 1866 29 March 1867	Arm	Worth 1, Co. List Aud. 6.1, p. 10
5	10 Oct 1866	Hand	Worth 3, Co. List
6	10 July 1866 30 Aug 1866 (2) 9 Nov 1866	Leg	Worth 3, form Jewett Invoices Aud. 6.1, p. 8 Worth 4, Co. List
7	13 May 1867	Arm	Aud. 6.1, p. 11
8	31 Oct 1866 (2) 2 May 1867	Leg	Jewett Invoices Aud. 6.1, p. 8 CW Military 41
9	2 May 1867	Arm	Aud. 6.1, p. 10
10	13 Sept 1866 1 Feb 1867 (2)	Leg	AG 58, p. 124 Jewett Invoices Aud. 6.1, p. 8
11	3 Dec 1866 11 Dec 1866 (2)	Leg	CW Military 41 Jewett Invoices Aud. 6.1, p. 9
12	21 May 1867 28 May 1867	Arm	CW Military 41 Aud. 6.1, p. 11
13	5 March 1866	Arm	Worth 2, Co. List
14	20 May 1867 21 May 1867	Leg	CW Military 41 Aud. 6.1, p. 12
15	28 July 1866 8 Aug 1866	Leg	CW Military 41 Worth 3, letter
16	10 Oct 1866	Leg	Worth 3, Co. List

	Claimant	County	Confederate Unit
1	Conrad, James	Forsyth	[Co. I and Band, 33rd NCT]
2	Conrad, L. L. (3)	Davidson	1st Co. D, 15th NCT (The Co. B recorded by Aud. is later designation—2nd Co. B, 49th NCT.)
3	Cook, J. H.	Davidson	Co. D, 13th NCT
4	Cook, James F. (2) (also Cooke)	Chatham	Co. A, 5th NCST
5	Cook, Lawson (2)	Mecklenburg	Co. C, 28th NCT
6	Cook, Levi H. (2) (also Cooke)	Chatham	Co. E, 5th NCST
7	Cook, Noah W. (3)	Cleveland	[Co. F], 55th NCT (erroneously listed as 35th NCT in Aud. 6.1, p. 9)
8	Corbitt, Dempsey	Pitt	Co. E, 27th NCT
9	Core, William (4)	Guilford	2nd Co. E, 2nd NCST
10	Corriker, Richard H. (2)	Rowan	Co. K, 57th NCT
11	Courtney, A. H. (3)	Caldwell	Co. F, 26th NCT
12	Courtney, John H. (3)	Buncombe	Co. I, 25th NCT
13	Covington, E. J.	Caswell	Co. A, 6th NCST
14	Covington, K. McR. (3)	Richmond	Co. E, 38th NCT
15	Covington, W. J. (2)	Rutherford	Co. E, 18th NCT

	Date	Limb	Location
1	8 March 1866	Leg	Worth 2, Co. List
2	18 July 1866 22 Dec 1866 (2)	Leg	Worth 3, form Jewett Invoices Aud. 6.1, p. 9
3	16 May 1867	Arm	Aud. 6.1, p. 11
4	5 Dec 1866 4 March 1867	Arm	Worth 4, Co. List Aud. 6.1, p. 9
5	4 June 1867 5 June 1867	Leg	CW Military 41 Aud. 6.1, p. 11
6	5 Dec 1866 4 March 1867	Arm	Worth 4, Co. List Aud. 6.1, p. 9
7	16 Nov 1866 20 Nov 1866 13 Dec 1867	Leg	CW Military 41 Aud. 6.1, p. 9 Aud. 6.1, p. 12
8	20 March 1867	Leg	Aud. 6.1, p. 8
9	no date 6 March 1867 11 March 1867 7 June 1867	Arm	Worth 8, Co. List CW Military 41 Aud. 6.1, p. 9 CW Military 41
10	23 April 1866 29 April 1867	Arm	CW Mil, Co. List Aud. 6.1, p. 10
11	12 July 1866 10 Jan 1867 (2)	Leg	Worth 3, form Jewett Invoices Aud. 6.1, p. 9
12	10 May 1866 15 Jan 1867 (2)	Leg	Worth 2, Co. List Jewett Invoices Aud. 6.1, p. 9
13	5 June 1867	Leg	Aud. 6.1, p. 11
14	28 June 1866 16 Oct 1866 (2)	Leg	CW Military 41 Jewett Invoices Aud. 6.1, p. 8
15	5 Jan 1867 (2)	Leg	Jewett Invoices Aud. 6.1, p. 9

	Claimant	County	Confederate Unit
1	Cowan, D. S.	Rowan	Co. B, 4th NCST
2	Cowan, James F.	Rowan	Co. B, 4th NCST
3	Cox, H. B. (3)	Moore	Co. D, 48th NCT
4	Cox, James H. (4)	Northampton	Co. H, 19th NCT (2nd NC Cav.)
5	Cox, John (3)	Yancey	Co. K, 15th NCT
6	Cox, Kerney	Mecklenburg	
7	Cox, William L.	Mecklenburg	Co. G, 34th NCT
8	Crabtree, John	Orange	Co. D, 1st NCST
9	Cranford, E. G. (3) *(see also Gorrell Cranford in CW Mil. 41)	Randolph, Montgomery, and Davidson	Co. F, 7th NCST
10	Cranford, Gorrell (3)	Davidson	
11	Crawford, Elias	Montgomery	Co. F, 44th NCT
12	Crawford, Joel T. (2)	Randolph	34th NCT
13	Creech, J. B.	Johnston	Co. I, 24th NCT
14	Crites, Sydney (2)	Yancey	[Co. C], 16th NCT
15	Cross, Silas (2)	Davidson	Co. B, 48th NCT
16	Crouch, Calvin (4)	Richmond and Robeson	Co. E, 38th NCT

	Date	Limb	Location
1	12 March 1867	Arm	Aud. 6.1, p. 10
2	22 March 1867	Arm	Aud. 6.1, p. 9
3	8 Aug 1866 9 July 1866 27 Sept 1866	Leg	AG 58, p. 59 Aud. 6.1, p. 8 Jewett Invoices
4	1 May 1866 30 July 1866 13 Nov 1866 (2)	Leg	Worth 2, Co. List Worth 3, form Jewett Invoices Aud. 6.1, p. 8
5	7 April 1866 15 Jan 1867 23 Jan 1867	Leg	Worth 2, Co. List CW Military 41 Aud. 6.1, p. 9
6	9 Nov 1866	Arm	Worth 4, Co. List
7	25 March 1867	Leg	Aud. 6.1, p. 10
8	11 April 1867	Arm	Aud. 6.1, p. 10
9	7 Dec 1866 17 July 1867 20 Feb 1867	Arm	Worth 4, letter CW Military 41* Aud. 6.1, p. 9
10	5 July 1867 17 July 1867 8 Aug 1867	Arm	CW Military 41 CW Military 41 CW Military 41
11	22 April 1867	Arm	Aud. 6.1, p. 10
12	1 Oct 1869 2 Oct 1869	Arm	TC $ Bk 4, p. 281 Aud. 6.1, p. 12
13	2 April 1867	Arm	Aud. 6.1, p. 10
14	7 April 1866 27 Feb 1867	Arm	Worth 2, Co. List Aud. 6.1, p. 9
15	5 June 1866 23 Feb 1867	Arm	CW Military 41 Aud. 6.1, p. 9
16	11 April 1866 3 Oct 1866 19 Dec 1866 (2)	Leg	Worth 2, Co. List CW Military 41 Jewett Invoices Aud. 6.1, p. 9

	Claimant	County	Confederate Unit
1	Crump, Thomas B. (3)	Anson	Co. C, 14th NCT
2	Cummings, Leonidas A. (4)	Rockingham	Co. F, 45th NCT
3	Currie, Daniel J. (4) (also J. D. Currie)	Robeson	Co. D, 51st NCT
4	Curtis, William (2)	Caldwell	Co. F, 26th NCT
5	Dail, Arthur (2)	Greene	Co. K, 33rd NCT
6	Dale, John H. (4)	McDowell	Co. B, 22nd NCT
7	Daniel, D. A. (2)	Alexander	Co. I, 37th NCT
8	Darden, A. L. (2)	Greene	Co. F, 61st NCT (incorrectly reported as 21st NCT on invoice)
9	Dare, Arthur	Greene	Co. K, 33rd NCT
10	Davenport, James A. (3)	Gaston	Co. M, 16th NCT
11	Davenport, William C.	Pitt	Co. B, 33rd NCT
12	David, John W.	Gaston	Co. K, 37th NCT
13	Davidson, Edward F. (2)	Mecklenburg	Co. E, 35th NCT
14	Davidson, J. P. A.	Mecklenburg	Co. K, 45th NCT
15	Davis, ————	Randolph	

	Date	Limb	Location
1	26 April 1867 20 May 1867 (2)	Arm	Worth 5, letter Jewett Invoices Aud. 6.1, p. 11
2	11 May 1867 15 May 1867 27 May 1867 19 June 1867	Arm	CW Military 41 Aud. 6.1, p. 11 CW Military 41 CW Military 41
3	3 July 1866 10 Oct 1866 31 Oct 1866 (2)	Leg	Worth 3, form Worth 3, Co. List Jewett Invoices Aud. 6.1, p. 8
4	1 March 1867 (2)	Arm	CW Military 41 Aud. 6.1, p. 9
5	21 Feb 1866 20 March 1867	Arm	Worth 1, Co. List CW Military 41
6	31 May 1866 10 Dec 1866 20 Dec 1866 (2)	Leg	Worth 2, Co. List Worth 4, letter Worth 4, letter Aud. 6.1, p. 13
7	1 March 1867 (2)	Leg	CW Military 41 Aud. 6.1, p. 13
8	25 Sept 1866 26 Sept 1866	Foot	Aud. 6.1, p. 13 Jewett Invoices
9	23 March 1867	Arm	Aud. 6.1, p. 14
10	no date 28 Sept 1867 2 Oct 1867	Arm	Worth 8, Co. List CW Military 41 Aud. 6.1, p. 15
11	4 May 1867	Arm	Aud. 6.1, p. 4
12	8 Nov 1866	Leg	Aud. 6.1, p. 13
13	1 Feb 1868 10 Feb 1868	Arm	CW Military 41 Aud. 6.1, p. 15
14	11 April 1867	Arm	Aud. 6.1, p. 15
15	29 Oct 1866	Leg	Worth 3, Co. List

	Claimant	County	Confederate Unit
1	Davis, David D. (3)	Rowan and Stanly	Co. K, 28th NCT
2	Davis, E. Hayne (2)	Iredell	A.A.A. & I.G. of Johnston's Brigade
3	Davis, E. M.	Anson	Co. K, 26th NCT
4	Davis, Elijah (5)	Wilkes	Co. F, 52nd NCT
5	Davis, George P. (2)	Cleveland	Co. C, 55th NCT
6	Davis, H. E.	Iredell	
7	Davis, Hampton (4)	Mississippi, then Anson	Co. I, 17th NCT
8	Davis, Haywood L. (5)	Wayne	Co. G, 47th NCT
9	Davis, J. L. (2)	Randolph	Co. G, 46th NCT
10	Davis, J. P.	Cleveland	Co. C, 55th NCT
11	Davis, J. W.		Co. K, 37th NCT
12	Davis, J. W.	Gaston	
13	Davis, James L. G. (3)	Martin	Co. G, 17th NCT
14	Davis, John H.	Davidson	Co. A, 6th NCST
15	Davis, M. T.	Onslow	Co. A, 33rd NCT

	Date	Limb	Location
1	24 Feb 1866 26 July 1866 (2)	Leg	Worth 1, Co. List Jewett Invoices Aud. 6.1, p. 13
2	13 March 1867 14 March 1867	Arm	CW Military 41 Aud. 6.1, p. 14
3	13 April 1867	Arm	Aud. 6.1, p. 14
4	11 April 1866 24 Aug 1866 (2) 1 Nov 1866 May 1867	Leg	Worth 2, Co. List CW Military 41 Aud. 6.1, p. 14 Worth 4, Co. List Jewett Invoices
5	no date 12 March 1867	Arm	Worth 8, Co. List CW Military 41
6	3 April 1866	Arm	Worth 2, Co. List
7	17 June 1867 25 Oct 1867 9 Aug 1867 17 Oct 1867	Leg	Worth 6, form Worth 7, receipt Aud. 6.1, p. 14 CW Military 41
8	18 April 1868 20 April 1868 4 May 1868 5 May 1868 no date	Arm	CW Military 41 TC $ Bk 4, p. 89 Aud. 6.1, p. 15 CW Military 41 CW Military 41
9	1 June 1866 (2)	Leg	Jewett Invoices Aud. 6.1, p. 13
10	16 March 1867	Arm	Aud. 6.1, p. 14
11	8 Nov 1866	Leg	Jewett Invoices
12	no date	Leg	Worth 8, Co. List
13	4 July 1866 10 July 1866 21 Sept 1867	Leg	Worth 3, form Worth 3, letter Aud. 6.1, p. 15
14	4 March 1867	Arm	Aud. 6.1, p. 14
15	8 April 1867	Arm	Aud. 6.1, p. 14

	Claimant	County	Confederate Unit
1	Davis, S. D. (3)	Cleveland	Co. B, 34th NCT
2	Davis, Solomon (3)	Madison	[Co. H, 2nd Bn. NC Inf.]
3	Davis, Thomas (2)	Cleveland	Co. B, 23rd NCT
4	Davis, Thomas E.	Chatham	Co. A, 26th NCT
5	Day, Carter (4)	Person	Co. E, 35th NCT
6	Day, John B. (4)	Person	Co. E, 15th NCT
7	Deal, Elkanah (4)	Catawba	Co. A, 12th NCT
8	Deal, R. A. (2)	Iredell	Co. A, 33rd NCT
9	Dean, B. H.	Johnston	Co. C, 5th NCST
10	DeArmond, James B. (5) (also Dearmon)	Mecklenburg	Co. F, 49th NCT
11	Delean, Alben (2) (also Albert DeLane)	Lincoln	Co. D, 7th NCST
12	Dellinger, Philip (5) (also Delinger)	Moore and Gaston	Co. I, 11th NCT

	Date	Limb	Location
1	27 Nov 1866 31 Dec 1866 (2)	Leg	CW Military 41 Jewett Invoices Aud. 6.1, p. 13
2	1 June 1868 3 June 1868 (2)	Arm	CW Military 41 TC $ Bk 4, p. 93 Aud. 6.1, p. 15
3	no date 8 April 1867	Arm	Worth 8, Co. List Aud. 6.1, p. 14
4	21 Feb 1867	Arm	Aud. 6.1, p. 14
5	6 June 1866 4 Sept 1866 (2) 27 Nov 1866	Leg	Worth 3, form Jewett Invoices Aud. 6.1, p. 13 Worth 4, Co. List
6	26 May 1866 13 Nov 1866 23 Nov 1866 27 Nov 1866	Leg	Worth 2, form Aud. 6.1, p. 13 Jewett Invoices Worth 4, Co. List
7	11 March 1868 12 March 1868 (3)	Arm	Worth 8, form Worth 8, letter (2) Aud. 6.1, p. 15
8	1 April 1867 3 April 1867	Arm	CW Military 41 Aud. 6.1, p. 14
9	21 Aug 1867	Leg	Aud. 6.1, p. 14
10	12 June 1866 18 Oct 1866 25 Oct 1866 26 Oct 1866 9 Nov 1866	Leg	Worth 3, form AG 58, p. 186 Aud. 6.1, p. 13 Jewett Invoices Worth 4, Co. List
11	25 March 1867 10 April 1867	Arm	CW Military 41 Aud. 6.1, p. 14
12	no date 10 Aug 1866 14 Aug 1866 (2) 20 Jan 1868	Leg	Worth 8, Co. List AG 58, p. 73 Jewett Invoices Aud. 6.1, p. 13 CW Military 41

	Claimant	County	Confederate Unit
1	Dent, A. T. (7)	Granville	Co. I, 55th NCT
2	Denton, James (4)	Edgecombe	Co. B, 33rd NCT
3	Denton, John B.	Franklin	Co. K, 12th NCT
4	Depriest, Jesse R. (3) (also Dupriest)	Rutherford	Co. G, 16th NCT
5	Derr, Andrew (2)	Gaston	Co. C, 37th NCT
6	Dickens, Elijah	Wayne	Co. I, 35th NCT
7	Dickey, James A.	Alamance	Co. E, 13th NCT
8	Dickey, James M.	Alamance	
9	Dills, A. M. (3)	Jackson	Co. G, 69th NCT
10	Dixon, M. L.	Rowan	Co. I, 22nd NCT
11	Dixon, Warren (3)	Person	Co. E, 35th NCT
12	Dockery, _____	Halifax	
13	Dodson, George W. (3)	Stokes	Co. H, 22nd NCT
14	Dorsey, E. W. (2)	Burke	Co. B., 11th NCT

	Date	Limb	Location
1	12 March 1866 10 Aug 1866 13 Aug 1866 15 Aug 1866 25 Sept 1866 27 Oct 1866 (2)	Leg and Arm	Worth 2, Co. List Worth 3, letter AG 58, p. 74 Worth 3, letter CW Military 41 Jewett Invoices Aud. 6.1, p. 13
2	6 Aug 1867 7 Aug 1867 10 Aug 1867 13 Aug 1867	Arm	CW Military 41 Aud. 6.1, p. 14 CW Military 41 CW Military 41
3	15 Aug 1867	Arm	Aud. 6.1, p. 14
4	18 Jan 1867 13 Feb 1867 May 1867	Leg	CW Military 41 Aud. 6.1, p. 13 Jewett Invoices
5	12 Sept 1866 (2)	Leg	Aud. 6.1, p. 13 Jewett Invoices
6	22 Feb 1867	Arm	Aud. 6.1, p. 14
7	18 April 1867	Arm	Aud. 6.1, p. 14
8	10 March 1866	Arm	Worth 2, Co. List
9	3 Nov 1866 27 Nov 1866 (2)	Leg	CW Military 41 Jewett Invoices Aud. 6.1, p. 13
10	19 March 1867	Arm	Aud. 6.1, p. 14
11	27 Nov 1866 23 Aug 1867 (2)	Leg	Worth 4, Co. List CW Military 41 Aud. 6.1, p. 15
12	5 March 1866	Arm	Worth 2, Co. List
13	10 Jan 1867 (2) 10 June 1867	Leg	Jewett Invoices Aud. 6.1, p. 13 CW Military 41
14	30 June 1866 18 Aug 1866	Leg	Worth 3, form Jewett Invoices

	Claimant	County	Confederate Unit
1	Douglass, A.	Yadkin	Co. F, 28th NCT
2	Douglass, William H. H. (4)	Hyde	Co. F, 33rd NCT
3	Dowdy, Archibald	Moore	Co. C, 35th NCT
4	Downs, James S. (6) (also Downes)	Caldwell and Alexander	Co. I, 26th NCT
5	Driver, John E. T. (2)	Davie	Co. F, 13th NCT
6	Drum, David J. (4)	Catawba	Co. C, 28th NCT
7	Dudley, Joseph (2)	Bertie	
8	Dukes, Thomas (5)	Northampton	Co. D, 59th NCT (4th NC Cav.)
9	Duncan, G. Wesley (7) (also erroneously given as J. Wesley Duncan) (Wesley returned his artificial leg in 1869.)	Wilkes and Alleghany	Co. D, 33rd NCT (Invoice erroneously indicates Co. B.)
10	Dunn, Bennett (3)	Pitt	Co. E, 3rd NCST

	Date	Limb	Location
1	27 March 1867	Arm	Aud. 6.1, p. 14
2	31 Oct 1867 7 Nov 1867 25 Nov 1867 10 Dec 1867	Leg	Worth 7, letter Worth 7, letter Aud. 6.1, p. 13 CW Military 41
3	15 April 1867	Arm	Aud. 6.1, p. 14
4	7 July 1866 5 Oct 1866 11 Oct 1866 (2) 1 Jan 1867 22 Feb 1868	Leg	Worth 3, form AG 58, p. 56 Jewett Invoices CW Military 41 Aud. 6.1, p. 13
5	22 Jan 1868 (2)	Hand	CW Military 41 Aud. 6.1, p. 15
6	25 Feb 1866 26 Nov 1866 4 Jan 1867 (2)	Leg	Worth 1, Co. List CW Military 41 Jewett Invoices Aud. 6.1, p. 13
7	27 Feb 1867 (2)	Arm	CW Military 41 Aud. 6.1, p. 14
8	1 May 1866 2 Aug 1866 27 Nov 1866 (2) 2 Jan 1868	Leg	Worth 2, Co. List Worth 3, form Jewett Invoices Aud. 6.1, p. 13 CW Military 41
9	11 April 1866 24 Aug 1866 1 Nov 1866 11 Feb 1867 (2) 12 June 1869 (2)	Leg	Worth 2, Co. List Worth 3, form Worth 4, Co. List Jewett Invoices Aud. 6.1, p. 13 TC $ Bk 4, p. 255 Aud. 6.1, p. 15
10	24 Aug 1866 30 Oct 1866 (2)	Leg	AG 58, p. 96 Jewett Invoices Aud. 6.1, p. 13

	Claimant	County	Confederate Unit
1	Dunn, Lemon (4) (name verified on 1870 census)	Pitt	Co. E, 43rd NCT
2	Dunn, Sidney M., Lt. (4)	Wake	[Co. A], 10th NCST (1st NC Arty.)
3	Dunning, James William (2)	Hertford	Co. I, 4th NCST
4	Dupree, John Q. (2)	Johnston	Co. E, 24th NCT
5	Dupree, Quinton	Johnston	
6	Dupriest—see Depriest		
7	Durham, Benjamin	Cleveland	[Co. I], 38th NCT
8	Eagle, Samuel (2)	Cabarrus	Co. A, 20th NCT
9	Eakes, Albert (3) (also Eaks)	Granville	Co. K, 55th NCT
10	Eakes, Madison (6)	Granville	Co. I, 23rd NCT (leg returned in 1870)
11	Earney, A. B. (3) (also Arney)	Gaston	Co. H, 52nd NCT
12	Earnheardt, T. M.	Rowan	Rowan Artillery [Co. D, 10th NCST (1st NC Arty.)]
13	Eason, William	Union	[Co. I, 53rd NCT]
14	Edge, Leonard (3) (also Lenon Edge)	Bladen	[Co. F, 24th NCT]
15	Edwards, A. (2)	Mecklenburg	

	Date	Limb	Location
1	18 May 1867 23 May 1867 12 July 1867 23 July 1867	Arm	CW Military 41 Aud. 6.1, p. 14 CW Military 41 CW Military 41
2	no date 8 Aug 1866 10 Aug 1866 (2)	Leg	CW Mil, Co. List AG 58, p. 56 Jewett Invoices Aud. 6.1, p. 13
3	1 March 1867 (2)	Arm	CW Military 41 Aud. 6.1, p. 14
4	25 July 1866 (2)	Leg	Jewett Invoices Aud. 6.1, p. 13
5	5 March 1866	Leg	Worth 2, Co. List
6			
7	27 Feb 1867	Arm	Aud. 6.1, p. 14
8	20 Dec 1866 21 Dec 1866	Leg	Worth 4, letter Aud. 6.1, p. 16
9	12 March 1866 13 April 1867 28 May 1867	Arm	Worth 2, Co. List CW Military 41 Aud. 6.1, p. 16
10	12 March 1866 14 June 1866 7 Aug 1866 (2) 6 April 1870 (2)	Leg	Worth 2, Co. List Worth 3, form Jewett Invoices Aud. 6.1, p. 16 TC $ Bk 4, p. 385 Aud. 6.1, p. 15
11	10 July 1866 2 May 1867 (2)	Leg	Worth 3, letter Jewett Invoices Aud. 6.1, p. 16
12	18 March 1867	Arm	Aud. 6.1, p. 16
13	22 Oct 1866	Leg	Worth 3, Co. List
14	10 April 1866 26 Feb 1867 (2)	Arm	Worth 2, Co. List CW Military 41 Aud. 6.1, p. 16
15	12 Oct 1866 18 Oct 1866		AG 58, p. 168 AG 58, p. 186

	Claimant	County	Confederate Unit
1	Edwards, Adolphus (2)	Lincoln	Co. C, 28th NCT (erroneously reported as Co. H in Aud.)
2	Edwards, Edward J.	Cumberland	Co. C, 3rd NCST
3	Edwards, Gilford (2)	Columbus	Co. C, 20th NCT
4	Edwards, William (2)	Yancey	
5	Eidson, M. F.	Iredell	Co. C, 48th NCT
6	Eller, Jacob (2)	Ashe	Co. L, 58th NCT
7	Eller, Samuel (3)	Rowan	Co. H, 23rd NCT
8	Ellis, James	Orange	Co. A, 24th NCT
9	Ellis, Jasper (2)	Wake	Co. E, 14th NCT
10	Ellis, Joseph (2)	Gates	Co. G, 52nd NCT
11	Ellis, William T. (2)	Onslow	Co. B, 24th NCT
12	Ennett, John (2) (also Ennitt)	Pasquotank	Co. C, 56th NCT
13	Ennis, John A. (2)	Harnett	Co. K, 3rd NCST
14	Eskridge, R. Calvin (2)	Cleveland	Co. C, 55th NCT
15	Eskridge, W. H. H. (2)	Cleveland	Co. E, 12th NCT
16	Essick, Jacob	Davidson	Co. K, 28th NCT
17	Estis, J. L. G. (2)	Caldwell	Co. F, 26th NCT

	Date	Limb	Location
1	23 Nov 1866 (2)	Leg	Jewett Invoices Aud. 6.1, p. 16
2	30 May 1867 1 June 1867	Arm	CW Military 41 Aud. 6.1, p. 16
3	12 Jan 1867 (2)	Leg	Jewett Invoices Aud. 6.1, p. 16
4	6 Nov 1867 13 Nov 1867	Legs	Worth 7, letter Aud. 6.1, p. 15
5	12 March 1867	Leg	Aud. 6.1, p. 16
6	25 May 1868 8 July 1868	Arm	CW Military 41 TC $ Bk 4, p. 99
7	23 April 1866 3 July 1866 (2)	Leg	CW Mil, Co. List Jewett Invoices Aud. 6.1, p. 16
8	2 May 1867	Arm	Aud. 6.1, p. 15
9	29 May 1867 30 May 1867	Hand	CW Military 41 Aud. 6.1, p. 16
10	9 June 1866 7 Nov 1866	Leg	Worth 3, form Aud. 6.1, p. 16
11	18 Dec 1866 21 Dec 1866	Leg	Worth 4, letter Aud. 6.1, p. 16
12	31 July 1866 (2)	Leg	Aud. 6.1, p. 16 Jewett Invoices
13	1 Feb 1869 (2)	Arm	TC $ Bk 4, p. 195 Aud. 6.1, p. 15
14	no date 16 March 1867	Arm	Worth 8, Co. List Aud. 6.1, p. 16
15	no date 27 Feb 1867	Arm	Worth 8, Co. List Aud. 6.1, p. 16
16	17 April 1867	Arm	Aud. 6.1, p. 16
17	1 March 1867 (2)	Arm	CW Military 41 Aud. 6.1, p. 16

	Claimant	County	Confederate Unit
1	Estis, L. E.	Wake	Co. E, 47th NCT
2	Ettres, Henry	Cleveland	Co. G, 49th NCT
3	Eudy, W. H. (2)	Stanly	Co. F, 5th NCST
4	Evans, Jefferson G. (3)	Guilford	Co. D, 1st NCST
5	Evans, John W. (2)	Caswell	Co. H, 6th NCST
6	Everitt, Thomas J.	Onslow	Co. E, 3rd NCST
7	Ezzell, Joseph C. (5) *(see also Walter R. Bell in CW Military 41)	Duplin	Co. B, 51st NCT
8	Falkner, John W.	Warren	Co. C, 46th NCT
9	Falls, Joseph O. (3)	Cleveland	Co. D, 14th NCT
10	Farmer, B. D. (2)	Wilson	Co. C, 43rd NCT
11	Farmer, J. C. (2)	Wilson	Co. F, 4th NCST
12	Farobee, B. L.	Davidson	Co. A, 21st NCT
13	Farthing, Robert	Watauga	Co. E, 37th NCT
14	Faucette, William F. (2)	Alamance	Co. C, 13th NCT
15	Faulk, Richard (2)	Robeson	[Co. C, 20th NCT]
16	Faulkner, James (2)	Warren	Co. D, 8th NCST
17	Fenton, Edmund F. (2) (also incorrectly given as Edward F. Fenton)	Anson	[Co. C, 14th NCT]

	Date	Limb	Location
1	25 May 1867	Hand	CW Military 41
2	8 April 1867	Arm	Aud. 6.1, p. 16
3	31 May 1867 (2)	Arm	CW Military 41 Aud. 6.1, p. 16
4	14 March 1867 no date (2)	Arm	Aud. 6.1, p. 16 Worth 8, Co. List and City List
5	20 Feb 1866 5 July 1867	Arm	Worth 1, Co. List Aud. 6.1, p. 16
6	10 Sept 1867	Arm	Aud. 6.1, p. 16
7	19 April 1866 18 March 1867 22 March 1867 30 March 1867 10 April 1867	Arm	CW Mil, Co. List CW Military 41* Aud. 6.1, p. 16 CW Military 41 CW Military 41
8	1 Aug 1867	Arm	Aud. 6.1, p. 18
9	no date 12 March 1867 16 March 1867	Arm	Worth 8, Co. List CW Military 41 Aud. 6.1, p. 17
10	31 July 1867 (2)	Arm	CW Military 41 Aud. 6.1, p. 18
11	31 July 1867 (2)	Arm	CW Military 41 Aud. 6.1, p. 18
12	3 June 1866	Leg	Aud. 6.1, p. 18
13	28 Feb 1867	Arm	Aud. 6.1, p. 17
14	10 March 1866 18 March 1867	Arm	Worth 2, Co. List Aud. 6.1, p. 17
15	21 Feb 1866 10 Oct 1866	Arm	Worth 1, Co. List Worth 3, Co. List
16	16 Oct 1866 (2)	Leg	Jewett Invoices Aud. 6.1, p. 17
17	23 March 1867 1 April 1867	Arm	CW Military 41 Aud. 6.1, p. 17

	Claimant	County	Confederate Unit
1	Ferebee, Joseph H. (3) (also Farobee)	Davie	Co. B, 19th Va.
2	Fergerson, W. R. (2) (also Ferguson)	Wake	
3	Ferguson, Simon (3) (also Simeon Furguson)	Cleveland	Co. D, 14th NCT
4	Fergusson, William R. (6) (also Furgesson) (1869 is probably return of leg for $50 commutation.)	Wilkes	Co. A, 37th NCT
5	Ferrell, Francis M. (2)	Wake	Co. D, 30th NCT
6	Ferrell, W. W.	Wake	Co. G, 7th NCST
7	Fesperman, W. C. (2)	Rowan	Co. F, 7th NCST
8	Fields, Bartholomew (3)	Lenoir	Co. C, 27th NCT
9	Fields, James N.	Sampson	Co. E, 26th NCT
10	Fields, Noah	Chatham	
11	Fink, Reuben P. (2)	Cabarrus	Co. G, 7th NCST
12	Fisher, Julius A. (2)	Stanly	Co. B, 57th NCT
13	Fleming, George H. (2)	Warren	Co. C, 46th NCT
14	Floyd, R. G. (3) (also R. C.)	Jackson	Thomas's Legion 69th NCT

	Date	Limb	Location
1	1 June 1866 20 Dec 1867 (2)	Arm	Worth 3, form CW Military 41 Aud. 6.1, p. 18
2	6 Oct 1866 2 Nov 1866	Leg	AG 58, p. 156 CW Military 41
3	no date 1 Dec 1866 11 Dec 1866	Leg	Worth 8, Co. List CW Military 41 Aud. 6.1, p. 17
4	11 April 1866 24 Aug 1866 17 Oct 1866 (2) 1 Nov 1866 26 April 1869	Leg	Worth 2, Co. List Worth 3, form Jewett Invoices Aud. 6.1, p. 17 Worth 4, Co. List TC $ Bk 4, p. 391
5	no date 8 March 1867	Arm	CW Mil, Co. List Aud. 6.1, p. 17
6	1 May 1867	Arm	Aud. 6.1, p. 18
7	6 July 1866 (2)	Leg	Aud. 6.1, p. 18 Jewett Invoices
8	20 March 1866 2 Oct 1866 (2)	Leg	Worth 2, Co. List Jewett Invoices Aud. 6.1, p. 17
9	22 April 1867	Arm	Aud. 6.1, p. 17
10	5 Dec 1866	Arm	Worth 4, Co. List
11	26 March 1866 6 April 1867	Arm	Worth 2, Co. List Aud. 6.1, p. 17
12	30 April 1867 4 May 1867	Leg	CW Military 41 Aud. 6.1, p. 18
13	20 June 1867 (2)	Arm	CW Military 41 Aud. 6.1, p. 18
14	16 Nov 1866 21 Dec 1866 (2)	Legs	CW Military 41 Jewett Invoices Aud. 6.1, p. 17

	Claimant	County	Confederate Unit
1	Fonville, B. F. (3)	Alamance	Co. K, 6th NCST
2	Ford, James A. (4)	Gaston	Co. H, 23rd NCT
3	Forester, Manly (3) (also Foister)	Chatham	Co. E, 26th NCT
4	Forrest, Calvin (2)	Greene	Co. G, 8th NCST
5	Forrest, T. F. (2)	Stanly	Co. H, 14th NCT
6	Fose, John	Catawba	
7	Foster, John A. (3)	Cherokee and Wilkes	Co. F, 52nd NCT
8	Fowler, E. W. (2)	Columbus	Co. C, 18th NCT
9	Fowler, Leonard (2)	Rutherford	Co. I, 34th NCT
10	Fowler, R. Warren (3)	Guilford	[2nd] Co. E, 2nd NCST
11	Fowler, William H.	Cumberland	Co. D, 57th NCT
12	Fox, David (2)	Alexander	[Co. F, 37th NCT]
13	Fox, Henry (4)	Caldwell	Co. F, 22nd NCT
14	Fox, John (3)	Catawba	Co. F, 38th NCT

	Date	Limb	Location
1	10 March 1866 4 March 1867 14 March 1867	Arm	Worth 2, Co. List CW Military 41 Aud. 6.1, p. 17
2	no date 24 Aug 1866 14 Sept 1866 (2)	Leg	Worth 8, Co. List AG 58, p. 90 Jewett Invoices Aud. 6.1, p. 17
3	5 Dec 1866 28 March 1867 (2)	Leg	Worth 4, Co. List Jewett Invoices Aud. 6.1, p. 17
4	30 April 1867 4 May 1867	Eyes	CW Military 41 Aud. 6.1, p. 18
5	31 May 1867 7 June 1867	Leg	CW Military 41 Aud. 6.1, p. 18
6	24 Feb 1866	Arm	Worth 1, Co. List
7	29 Oct 1866 (2) 1 Nov 1866	Leg	Jewett Invoices Aud. 6.1, p. 17 Worth 4, Co. List
8	21 Dec 1866 (2)	Leg	Jewett Invoices Aud. 6.1, p. 17
9	11 Dec 1866 (2)	Leg	Jewett Invoices Aud. 6.1, p. 17
10	3 June 1867 no date (2)	Arm	Aud. 6.1, p. 18 Worth 8, Co. List and City List
11	5 July 1867	Arm	Aud. 6.1, p. 18
12	19 Jan 1867 9 Feb 1867	Foot	CW Military 41 Aud. 6.1, p. 17
13	16 July 1866 (2) 23 Jan 1867 (2)	Leg	Worth 3, form CW Military 41 Jewett Invoices Aud. 6.1, p. 17
14	1 May 1867 4 May 1867 6 May 1867	Arm	CW Military 41 Aud. 6.1, p. 18 CW Military 41

	Claimant	County	Confederate Unit
1	Foy, Solomon E. (2)	Gaston	Co. H, 49th NCT
2	Franklin, Jacob (3)	Cherokee	[Co. F, 39th NCT]
3	Frazier, Alex J. (2)	Guilford	Co. E, 22nd NCT
4	Frazier, Elijah (3)	Granville	Co. K, 55th NCT
5	Frazier, James R.	Randolph	Co. D, 44th Tenn.
6	Frazier, Rhodes M. (3)	Granville	Co. K, 55th NCT
7	Frazier, Thomas (3)	Granville	Co. I, 23rd NCT
8	Freeman, Reuben (3)	Montgomery	Co. F, 14th NCT
9	Freeman, W. H. (2)	Surry	
10	Fritchett, Daniel E. (2) (also Fitchett)	Guilford	
11	Fry, Calvin (2)	Stanly	Co. H, 14th NCT
12	Fry, J. Pinckney (4)	Catawba	[2nd] Co. B, 42nd NCT
13	Fulcher, Silas (2)	Craven	Co. F, 2nd NCST
14	Fulton, H. D. (3)	Cleveland	Co. G, 49th NCT

	Date	Limb	Location
1	no date 27 Feb 1867	Arm	Worth 8, Co. List Aud. 6.1, p. 17
2	20 July 1866 18 Aug 1867 19 Aug 1868	Leg	Worth 3, letter Aud. 6.1, p. 18 TC $ Bk 4, p. 111
3	no date 19 March 1867	Arm	Worth 8, Co. List Aud. 6.1, p. 17
4	12 March 1866 13 April 1867 28 May 1867	Arm	Worth 2, Co. List CW Military 41 Aud. 6.1, p. 18
5	28 Aug 1867	Leg	Aud. 6.1, p. 18
6	12 March 1866 10 April 1867 28 May 1867	Arm	Worth 2, Co. List CW Military 41 Aud. 6.1, p. 18
7	12 March 1866 13 April 1867 28 May 1867	Arm	Worth 2, Co. List Worth 5, letter Aud. 6.1, p. 18
8	no date 26 Nov 1867 1 Dec 1867	Leg	CW Military 41 Worth 7, letter Aud. 6.1, p. 18
9	26 May 1866 3 June 1866	Leg	Worth 2, letter Aud. 6.1, p. 18
10	23 Jan 1867 (2)	Leg	Jewett Invoices Aud. 6.1, p. 17
11	31 May 1867 (2)	Arm	CW Military 41 Aud. 6.1, p. 18
12	24 Feb 1866 16 April 1867 25 April 1867 1 May 1867	Arm	Worth 1, Co. List CW Mil, Co. List Aud. 6.1, p. 18 CW Military 41
13	8 Jan 1867 25 Jan 1867	Leg	Worth 4, letter Aud. 6.1, p. 17
14	16 April 1867 23 April 1867 27 May 1867	Leg	CW Military 41 Aud. 6.1, p. 17 CW Military 41

	Claimant	County	Confederate Unit
1	Fuqua, Quentin A.	Rockingham	Co. I, 13th NCT
2	Futrell, Bryan G. (2) (also erroneously listed as Bryant G. Futrell)	Northampton	[Co. B, 9th NCST (1st NC Cav.)]
3	Gadd, ————	Randolph	
4	Gadd, Armsted	Rowan	Co. H, 38th NCT
5	Gadd, James E.	Montgomery	Co. K, 26th NCT
6	Gaines, James L., Lt. Col. (2)	Buncombe	9th NCT (1st NC Cav.) [19th NCT (2nd NC Cav.)]
7	Gardner, John T. (2)	Bertie	Co. G, 32nd NCT
8	Gardner, Wilie (2) (also Garner, Wiley)	Johnston	Co. C, 5th NCST
9	Garner, Francis M. (4) (also Frank)	Duplin	Co. C, 51st NCT
10	Garner, James (3)	Johnston	Co. C, 5th NCST
11	Garrett, G. W. (4)	Gaston	Co. H, 23rd NCT
12	Garrison, D. B. (5)	Mecklenburg	C. S. Navy
13	Garvin, William C.	McDowell	[Co. B, 22nd NCT]
14	Gash, Joseph R. (2)	Henderson	Co. I, 16th NCT
15	Gaskins, Henry (3)	Craven	Latham's Arty. [1st Co. H, 40th NCT, (3rd NC Arty.)]

	Date	Limb	Location
1	16 May 1867	Leg	Aud. 6.1, p. 18
2	1 May 1866 17 Sept 1880	Arm	Worth 2, Co. List CW Military 41
3	29 Oct 1866	Arm	Worth 3, Co. List
4	2 Nov 1867	Arm	Aud. 6.1, p. 21
5	4 Nov 1867	Arm	Aud. 6.1, p. 21
6	30 March 1867 (2)	Arm	Jewett Invoices Aud. 6.1, p. 19
7	24 May 1867 4 June 1867	Arm	CW Military 41 Aud. 6.1, p. 21
8	1 April 1867 27 May 1867	Arm	CW Military 41 Aud. 6.1, p. 20
9	19 April 1866 22 Nov 1866 8 Jan 1867 (2)	Leg	CW Military 41 CW Mil, Co. List Jewett Invoices Aud. 6.1, p. 19
10	5 March 1866 19 June 1866 (2)	Leg	Worth 2, Co. List Jewett Invoices Aud. 6.1, p. 19
11	29 April 1867 4 July 1867 15 Aug 1867 30 Aug 1867	Arm	CW Military 41 CW Military 41 CW Military 41 CW Military 41
12	8 June 1866 30 July 1866 10 Aug 1866 30 Aug 1866 (2)	Foot	Worth 3, form Worth 3, letter AG 58, p. 80 Jewett Invoices Aud. 6.1, p. 19
13	31 May 1866	Hand	Worth 2, Co. List
14	16 April 1866 12 March 1867	Leg	Worth 2, Co. List Aud. 6.1, p. 20
15	27 Aug 1866 28 Feb 1867 (2)	Leg	Worth 3, form Jewett Invoices Aud. 6.1, p. 19

	Claimant	County	Confederate Unit
1	Gatlin, Francis P. (2)	Craven	Latham's Arty. [1st Co. H, 40th NCT, (3rd NC Arty.)]
2	Gause, James W. (5)	Bladen	Co. B, 18th NCT
3	Gay, Daniel O. (3)	Richmond	Co. E, 52nd NCT
4	Gibbons, C[ornelius] R.	Cleveland	[Co. F, 34th NCT]
5	Gibson, Thomas A. (2)	Mecklenburg	Co. C, 37th NCT
6	Gibson, William M. (2)	Caldwell	Co. I, 26th NCT
7	Gilbert, Joseph	Wake	Co. G, 7th NCST
8	Gilbert, Robert (4)	Lincoln	Co. K, 23rd NCT
9	Gillaspie, J. M.	Cleveland	Co. H, 28th NCT
10	Gladden, James (2)	Cleveland	Co. B, 49th NCT
11	Gladson, James (2)	Rowan	Co. D, 7th NCST
12	Gladson, William D. (4)	Pitt	Co. D, 44th NCT
13	Gleason, James	Rowan	[Co. D, 7th NCST]
14	Glen, Franklin	Mecklenburg	
15	Glenn, D. P.	Mecklenburg	Co. A, 11th NCT
16	Glenn, Wiley	Wake	Co. E, 47th NCT

	Date	Limb	Location
1	22 Aug 1866 15 Oct 1866	Leg	Worth 3, form Aud. 6.1, p. 19
2	10 April 1866 22 June 1866 9 Feb 1867 12 Feb 1867 13 Feb 1867	Leg	Worth 3, form Worth 2, Co. List CW Mil, Co. List Aud. 6.1, p. 19 Jewett Invoices
3	11 April 1866 21 Dec 1866 (2)	Leg	Worth 2, Co. List Jewett Invoices Aud. 6.1, p. 19
4	no date	Arm	Worth 8, Co. List
5	7 Jan 1868 (2)	Arm	CW Military 41 Aud. 6.1, p. 21
6	9 May 1868 (2)	Leg	Worth 8, letter Aud. 6.1, p. 1
7	22 May 1867	Arm	Aud. 6.1, p. 20
8	15 Sept 1866 18 Oct 1866 30 Oct 1866 (2)	Leg	Worth 3, letter AG 58, p. 180 Jewett Invoices Aud. 6.1, p. 19
9	8 April 1867	Arm	Aud. 6.1, p. 20
10	23 Nov 1866 29 Nov 1866	Leg	CW Military 41 Aud. 6.1, p. 19
11	21 Aug 1866 (2)	Foot	Jewett Invoices Aud. 6.1, p. 19
12	10 Dec 1866 (2) 1 May 1867 1 June 1867	Leg	Jewett Invoices Aud. 6.1, p. 19 CW Military 41 CW Military 41
13	23 April 1866	Foot	CW Mil, Co. List
14	9 Nov 1866	Arm	Worth 4, Co. List
15	29 March 1867	Arm	Aud. 6.1, p. 20
16	19 May 1867	Arm	Aud. 6.1, p. 20

	Claimant	County	Confederate Unit
1	Glisson, Henry J. (2)	Duplin	Co. C, 2nd NCST
2	Godfrey, Pleasant	Chatham	Co. E, 10th NCST (1st NC Arty.)
3	Godwin, James T.	Wilson	Co. A, 16th Bn. NC Cav.
4	Godwin, Sir William	Wake	Co. D, 26th NCT
5	Goforth, J. N. (2)	Iredell	Co. H, 4th NCST
6	Goins, Henry (2)	Burke	Co. E, 16th NCT
7	Goode, David P. (6)	Cleveland	Co. E, 12th NCT
8	Gooding, William B. (3)	McDowell	Co. K, 22nd NCT
9	Goodwin, J. P. (2)	Wake	Co. D, 31st NCT
10	Goodwin, J. R.	Harnett	Co. H, 20th NCT
11	Goodwin, Lewis (3)	Beaufort	Co. B, 40th NCT
12	Goodwin, Timothy	Moore	Co. C, 35th NCT
13	Gordon, Alston (2) (also Austin)	Haywood and Cleveland	Co. F, 25th NCT
14	Gordon, William W.	Guilford	
15	Gorrell, William M.	Guilford	Co. E, 29th Miss.
16	Goslin, Aug	Forsyth	
17	Goslin, L. A. (3)	Forsyth	Co. I, 33rd NCT

	Date	Limb	Location
1	26 Nov 1867 30 Nov 1867	Hand	CW Military 41 Aud. 6.1, p. 21
2	16 May 1867	Arm	Aud. 6.1, p. 20
3	15 May 1867	Arm	Aud. 6.1, p. 20
4	21 May 1867	Arm	Aud. 6.1, p. 20
5	20 March 1867 21 March 1867	Arm	CW Military 41 Aud. 6.1, p. 19
6	13 March 1867 18 March 1867	Arm	CW Military 41 Aud. 6.1, p. 20
7	no date 1 July 1866 20 July 1866 20 Nov 1866 19 Dec 1866 (2)	Leg	Worth 8, Co. List Worth 3, letter AG 58, p. 47 CW Military 41 Jewett Invoices Aud. 6.1, p. 19
8	31 May 1866 20 May 1867 1 June 1867	Arm	Worth 2, Co. List CW Military 41 Aud. 6.1, p. 20
9	2 March 1867 (2)	Arm	CW Military 41 Aud. 6.1, p. 19
10	17 April 1867	Leg	Aud. 6.1, p. 20
11	26 Sept 1866 26 April 1867 (2)	Arm	CW Military 41 Jewett Invoices Aud. 6.1, p. 20
12	23 April 1867	Arm	Aud. 6.1, p. 20
13	15 May 1866 27 Feb 1867	Leg	Worth 2, Co. List Aud. 6.1, p. 19
14	no date	Arm	Worth 8, City List
15	no date	Arm	Worth 8, Co. List
16	8 March 1866	Leg	Worth 2, Co. List
17	25 June 1866 4 July 1866 (2)	Leg	Worth 3, form Jewett Invoices Aud. 6.1, p. 19

	Claimant	County	Confederate Unit
1	Grady, John R. (2)	Anson	[Co. A, 23rd NCT]
2	Graham, Neill A.	Robeson	[Co. C, 3rd NCST]
3	Graham, William H.	Wake	Co. H, 26th NCT
4	Grant, Ichabod	Wayne	Co. C, 66th NCT
5	Graves, John C. (2)	Davie	Co. F, 13th NCT
6	Gray, Parrott M. (2)	Lenoir	Co. A, 40th NCT
7	Gray, William H. (3)	Guilford and Hyde	Co. F, 33rd NCT
8	Green, Exum (3)	Gates	Co. H, 5th NCST
9	Green, William R. (2)	Franklin	Co. I, 55th NCT
10	Greenwood, G. W. (2)	Surry	54th NCT
11	Greer—see Grier		
12	Greeson, David L. (3)	Guilford	Co. B, 45th NCT
13	Gregory, Jesse (2)	Macon	Co. B, 39th NCT
14	Gregory, John T. (2)	Sampson	Co. C, 3rd Ark.
15	Gregory, Nathaniel (4)	Rockingham	Co. K, 13th NCT
16	Grier, Vincent (5) (also Greer) (erroneously listed as Vinson Green in Aud.)	Wilkes	Co. G, 18th NCT

	Date	Limb	Location
1	26 April 1867 1 May 1867	Arm	Worth 5, letter Aud. 6.1, p. 20
2	10 Oct 1866	Arm	Worth 3, Co. List
3	14 May 1867	Arm	Aud. 6.1, p. 20
4	4 April 1867	Arm	Aud. 6.1, p. 20
5	13 March 1866 26 April 1867	Arm	Worth 2, Co. List Aud. 6.1, p. 20
6	20 March 1866 12 April 1867	Arm	Worth 2, Co. List Aud. 6.1, p. 2
7	5 Oct 1866 22 Oct 1866 (2)	Leg	AG 58, p. 149 Jewett Invoices Aud. 6.1, p. 21
8	20 Aug 1866 8 Nov 1866 (2)	Leg	Worth 3, form Jewett Invoices Aud. 6.1, p. 19
9	3 Jan 1867 (2)	Leg	Jewett Invoices Aud. 6.1, p. 19
10	23 Feb 1867 (2)	Arm	CW Military 41 Aud. 6.1, p. 21
11			
12	28 Feb 1867 no date (2)	Arm	Aud. 6.1, p. 19 Worth 8, Co. List and City List
13	2 Aug 1867 5 Aug 1867	Arm	Aud. 6.1, p. 21 CW Military 41
14	28 Aug 1866 29 Aug 1866	Leg	Worth 3, form Aud. 6.1, p. 19
15	12 March 1866 (2) 12 Oct 1866 (2)	Leg	CW Mil, Co. List AG 58, p. 167 Jewett Invoices Aud. 6.1, p. 19
16	11 April 1866 24 Aug 1866 1 Nov 1866 21 Jan 1867 (2)	Leg	Worth 2, Co. List Worth 3, form Worth 4, Co. List Jewett Invoices Aud. 6.1, p. 19

	Claimant	County	Confederate Unit
1	Griffin, George W.	Wilson	Capt. Bass's Co. [Co. D, 8th Bn. NC Partisan Rangers]
2	Griffin, James P. (4)	Union	Co. D, 37th NCT
3	Griffin, Vincent R.	Rockingham	Co. K, 5th NC Cav.
4	Grigg, Eli	Cleveland	[Co. K, 49th NCT]
5	Groner, H. L. (3)	Cabarrus	Co. A, 20th NCT
6	Grubb, Alex	Davidson	Co. A, 54th NCT
7	Gulledge, William D.	Anson	
8	Gunter, W. W.	Chatham	Co. G, 7th NCST
9	Gurley, William H. (4) (Invoices state that Gurley received a "support" and that the state was overcharged for it.)	Wayne	Co. D, 4th NCST
10	Hagler, James	Cabarrus	[Co. C, 33rd NCT]
11	Hahn, E. B.	Warren	Co. F, 8th NCST
12	Hahn, Samuel A.	Gaston	Co. B, 28th NCT
13	Hair, Daniel (2)	Harnett	Co. C, 36th NCT
14	Hall, A. W. (2)	Randolph	Co. B, 57th NCT
15	Hall, Calvin	Montgomery	Co. D, 44th NCT
16	Hall, James (3)	Stanly	Co. H, 14th NCT
17	Hall, James L.	Sampson	Co. D, 53rd NCT

	Date	Limb	Location
1	3 May 1867	Arm	Aud. 6.1, p. 20
2	22 Oct 1866 27 May 1867 1 June 1867 8 June 1867	Leg	Worth 3, Co. List CW Military 41 Aud. 6.1, p. 20 CW Military 41
3	3 May 1867	Arm	Aud. 6.1, p. 20
4	no date	Arm	Worth 8, Co. List
5	26 March 1866 6 Sept 1866 (2)	Leg	Worth 2, Co. List CW Military 41 Aud. 6.1, p. 19
6	4 March 1867	Arm	Aud. 6.1, p. 20
7	1 May 1867	Arm	Aud. 6.1, p. 20
8	24 May 1867	Arm	Aud. 6.1, p. 20
9	21 Jan 1867 2 Feb 1867 (2) Feb-March 1867	Leg	CW Military 41 Jewett Invoices Aud. 6.1, p. 19 Jewett Invoices
10	26 March 1866	Arm	Worth 2, Co. List
11	28 Aug 1867	Arm	Aud. 6.1, p. 25
12	27 Feb 1867	Arm	Aud. 6.1, p. 23
13	23 May 1867 25 May 1867	Arm	CW Military 41 Aud. 6.1, p. 25
14	11 Dec 1866 (2)	Leg	Jewett Invoices Aud. 6.1, p. 23
15	3 Feb 1868	Arm	Aud. 6.1, p. 26
16	24 Feb 1866 May 1867 no date	Leg	Worth 1, Co. List Jewett Invoices Aud. 6.1, p. 24
17	3 April 1867	Arm	Aud. 6.1, p. 24

	Claimant	County	Confederate Unit
1	Hall, Moses (2)	McDowell	Co. K, 60th NCT
2	Halsy, John (2)	Ashe	Co. K, 37th NCT
3	Ham, Jacob (2)	Ashe	Co. A, [9th NCST (1st NC Cav.)]
4	Ham, Stephen (3)	Harnett	Co. F, 15th NCT
5	Ham, Thomas (2)	Ashe	Co. A, 37th NCT
6	Hamilton, W. H.	Wake	Co. E, 14th NCT
7	Hampton, Wade	Yancey	[Co. D, 69th NCT (7th NC Cav.)]
8	Hamrick, A. L.	Cleveland	Co. D, 55th NCT
9	Hamrick, A. M.	Cleveland	Co. D, 55th NCT
10	Hamrick, H. G. (2)	Cleveland	Co. D, 55th NCT
11	Hancock, Noah (2)	Randolph	Co. F, 46th NCT
12	Hand, S. J.	Gaston	[Co. B, 28th NCT]
13	Hanna, R. Alexander (3)	Anson	Co. K, 26th NCT
14	Harbin, J. F. (3)	Iredell	Co. C, 4th NCST
15	Harbison, W. T. (3)	Burke	Co. B, 10th NCST (listed as Co. B, 11th NCT in *NCT Roster*)
16	Hardee, John L. (3)	Lenoir	Co. D, 66th NCT

	Date	Limb	Location
1	31 May 1866 7 May 1867	Arm	Worth 2, Co. List Aud. 6.1, p. 26
2	10 Dec 1867 (2)	Arm	CW Military 41 Aud. 6.1, p. 26
3	14 Oct 1868 9 Jan 1869	Arm	Aud 6.113 Aud. 6.1, p. 26
4	3 June 1867 8 June 1867 10 June 1867	Leg	CW Military 41 Aud. 6.1, p. 25 CW Military 41
5	8 Feb 1869 (2)	Arm	TC $ Bk 4, p. 197 Aud. 6.1, p. 26
6	4 March 1867	Eyes	Aud. 6.1, p. 23
7	28 Feb 1867	Arm	Aud. 6.1, p. 23
8	16 March 1867	Arm	Aud. 6.1, p. 23
9	12 March 1867	Arm	CW Military 41
10	12 March 1867 16 March 1867	Arm	CW Military 41 Aud. 6.1, p. 23
11	26 Feb 1868 (2)	Leg	Worth 8, letter Aud. 6.1, p. 26
12	no date	Arm	Worth 8, Co. List
13	8 June 1866 18 Jan 1867 (2)	Leg	Worth 3, form Jewett Invoices Aud. 6.1, p. 24
14	3 April 1866 21 Feb 1867 27 Feb 1867	Arm	Worth 2, Co. List CW Military 41 Aud. 6.1, p. 23
15	30 June 1866 6 Nov 1866 (2)	Leg	Worth 3, form Jewett Invoices Aud. 6.1, p. 22
16	20 March 1866 15 March 1867 19 March 1867	Arm	Worth 2, Co. List CW Military 41 Aud. 6.1, p. 24

	Claimant	County	Confederate Unit
1	Harden, Leander C. (2) (also Hartin)	Wilkes	
2	Hardin, Walter R. (4)	Cleveland	Co. C, 15th NCT
3	Hardison, Ira T. (3) *(see also James T. Brown in CW Mil. 41)	Martin	[Co. A], 17th NCT
4	Harp, William	Franklin	Co. I, 55th NCT
5	Harper, Robert H. (3)	Halifax	Co. F, 43rd NCT
6	Harrell, John B. (2)	Rutherford	Co. I, 56th NCT
7	Harrelson, J. B.	Columbus	Co. D, 20th NCT
8	Harrington, John	Alexander	Co. G, 37th NCT
9	Harris, B. F.	Montgomery	Co. C, 23rd NCT
10	Harry, William B. (4)	Mecklenburg	Co. B, 53rd NCT
11	Hart, A. C. (2)	Greene	[Co. B, 63rd NCT (5th NC Cav.)]
12	Hart, R. R.	Alexander	Co. B, 2nd NC Cav.
13	Hart, Richard A. (4)	Granville	Co. D, 12th NCT
14	Hart, Richard A. (2)	Wilson	
15	Harten, Bud	Wilkes	
16	Harten, L. C.	Wilkes	
17	Hartley, T. H.	Caldwell	Co. I, 26th NCT

	Date	Limb	Location
1	1 Nov 1866 19 Jan 1867	Arm	Worth 4, Co. List CW Military 41
2	no date 23 Nov 1866 20 Dec 1866 (2)	Leg	Worth 8, Co. List CW Military 41 Jewett Invoices Aud. 6.1, p. 24
3	24 Aug 1867 27 Sept 1867	Arm	CW Military 41* Aud. 6.1, p. 25
4	18 June 1867	Leg	CW Military 41
5	17 Sept 1867 6 Nov 1867 9 Nov 1867	Arm	CW Military 41 Aud. 6.1, p. 26 CW Military 41
6	23 July 1867 25 July 1867	Arm	Aud. 6.1, p. 25 CW Military 41
7	22 Feb 1867	Arm	Aud. 6.1, p. 23
8	20 Dec 1867	Leg	Aud. 6.1, p. 24
9	12 June 1867	Arm	Aud. 6.1, p. 25
10	18 June 1866 1 Aug 1866 (2) 9 Nov 1866	Leg	Worth 3, form Aud. 6.1, p. 22 Jewett Invoices Worth 4, Co. List
11	21 Feb 1866 15 April 1867	Arm	Worth 1, Co. List Aud. 6.1, p. 25
12	11 April 1867	Arm	Aud. 6.1, p. 25
13	12 March 1866 14 June 1866 19 June 1866 (2)	Leg	Worth 2, Co. List Worth 3, form Jewett Invoices Aud. 6.1, p. 22
14	26 June 1866 29 June 1866	Leg	CW Military 41 AG 58, p. 36
15	11 April 1866	Arm	Worth 2, Co. List
16	23 Feb 1867	Arm	Aud. 6.1, p. 26
17	13 May 1867	Arm	Aud. 6.1, p. 25

	Claimant	County	Confederate Unit
1	Hartmon, John H. (2)	Cleveland	Co. D, 2nd Jr. Res.
2	Harvell, James	Columbus	
3	Harvey, James	Columbus	Co. H, 18th NCT
4	Hass, S. A.	Mecklenburg	Co. C, 28th NCT
5	Hastings, Albert (2)	Macon	Co. H, 16th NCT
6	Hawes, R. J. T. (3)	Duplin	Co. A, 51st NCT
7	Hawk, Michael	Ashe	Co. A, 26th NCT
8	Hawkins, Edward	Cleveland	Co. G, 18th NCT
9	Hawkins, F. A. (4)	Mecklenburg	Co. B, 13th NCT
10	Hawkins, Francis (2)	Jones	Co. G, 2nd NCST
11	Hawkins, W. J.	Cleveland	Co. H, 28th NCT
12	Hawkins, William A.	Stokes	Co. L, 21st NCT
13	Hayes, Thomas (3)	Transylvania	Co E, 25th NCT
14	Hays, Josephus (3)	Gates	Co. B, 5th NCST
15	Heart, A. J.	Henderson	
16	Heathcock, Jesse	Stanly	Co. H, 14th NCT
17	Heavner, L. J. (2)	Gaston	Co. I, 11th NCT

	Date	Limb	Location
1	2 Oct 1867 (2)	Hand	CW Military 41 Aud. 6.1, p. 25
2	26 Feb 1867	Arms	CW Military 41
3	26 Feb 1867	Arm	Aud. 6.1, p. 23
4	5 April 1867	Arm	Aud. 6.1, p. 24
5	9 July 1867 22 Aug 1867	Leg	CW Military 41 Aud. 6.1, p. 25
6	19 April 1866 28 Nov 1866 (2)	Leg	CW Mil, Co. List Jewett Invoices Aud. 6.1, p. 22
7	26 Feb 1867	Arm	CW Military 41
8	8 April 1867	Arm	Aud. 6.1, p. 24
9	19 June 1866 18 Aug 1866 (2) 9 Nov 1866	Leg	Worth 3, form Jewett Invoices Aud. 6.1, p. 22 Worth 4, Co. List
10	27 Sept 1867 (2)	Arm	CW Military 41 Aud. 6.1, p. 26
11	8 April 1867	Arm	Aud. 6.1, p. 24
12	25 March 1867	Arm	Aud. 6.1, p. 24
13	30 March 1867 5 April 1867 16 April 1867	Leg	Worth 4, letter CW Military 41 Aud. 6.1, p. 24
14	22 Aug 1866 14 Nov 1866 (2)	Leg	Worth 3, form Jewett Invoices Aud. 6.1, p. 22
15	16 April 1866	Leg	Worth 2, Co. List
16	18 May 1867	Leg	Aud. 6.1, p. 25
17	no date 5 April 1867	Arm	Worth 8, Co. List Aud. 6.1, p. 24

	Claimant	County	Confederate Unit
1	Hedgepeth, John Thomas (6)	Robeson	Co. A, 31st NCT
2	Hedrick, Andrew (3) (also Heedick)	Lincoln	Co. B, 23rd NCT
3	Hege, Alexander	Davidson	Co. K, 15th NCT
4	Hellin, John T.	Pitt	Co. E, 55th NCT
5	Helms, Alexander (2)	Lincoln	Co. E, 34th NCT (CW Mil. 41 erroneously indicates 43rd NCT.)
6	Helms, C. A. (4)	Union	Co. B, 43rd NCT
7	Helsebach, Gaston J. (4) (also Helesobeck)	Forsyth	Co. C, 33rd NCT
8	Hembree, James W. (3)	Buncombe	Co. F, 16th NCT
9	Henderson, A. E. (3)	Granville	Co. B, 12th NCT
10	Henderson, David J. (3)	Onslow	Co. A, 35th NCT
11	Hendrick, William D. (2)	Cleveland	Co. D, 55th NCT
12	Hennessa, E. A. (3)	Burke	Co. D, 11th NCT

	Date	Limb	Location
1	21 Feb 1866 14 Aug 1866 Sept 1866 2 Oct 1866 (2) 10 Oct 1866	Leg	Worth 1, Co. List Worth 3, form AG 58, p. 118 Jewett Invoices Aud. 6.1, p. 22 Worth 3, Co. List
2	21 March 1867 10 April 1867 15 April 1867	Arm	CW Military 41 Aud. 6.1, p. 25 CW Military 41
3	23 April 1867	Eyes	Aud. 6.1, p. 26
4	7 Aug 1866	Leg	Aud. 6.1, p. 22
5	23 March 1867 10 April 1867	Arm	CW Military 41 Aud. 6.1, p. 24
6	29 May 1866 2 Aug 1866 27 Aug 1866 31 Aug 1866	Leg	Worth 2, form Aud. 6.1, p. 22 AG 58, p. 101 Jewett Invoices
7	8 March 1866 23 June 1866 27 July 1866 (2)	Leg	Worth 2, Co. List Worth 3, form Jewett Invoices Aud. 6.1, p. 22
8	10 May 1866 15 Dec 1866 (2)	Leg	Worth 2, Co. List Jewett Invoices Aud. 6.1, p. 24
9	12 March 1866 20 June 1866 10 Jan 1867	Leg	Worth 2, Co. List CW Military 41 Aud. 6.1, p. 24
10	3 Dec 1866 12 Jan 1867 (2)	Leg	CW Military 41 Jewett Invoices Aud. 6.1, p. 24
11	3 Dec 1866 10 Jan 1867	Leg	CW Military 41 Jewett Invoices
12	6 April 1867 10 April 1867	Arm	CW Military 41 (2) Aud. 6.1, p. 24

	Claimant	County	Confederate Unit
1	Hepler, S. J. (3)	Davidson	Co. B, 14th NCT
2	Herndon, William	Orange	Co. F, 1st NCST
3	Herrin, Eli R. (3) (also Herron)	Stanly	Co. K, 28th NCT
4	Herrin, Julius	Stanly	Co. H, 42nd NCT
5	Hicks, John	Watauga	Co. D, 13th NCT
6	Higgins, Griggs (3)	Alleghany	Co. C, 63rd Va.
7	Hill, Robert (4)	Lenoir	Co. E, 66th NCT
8	Hines, G. D. (2)	Guilford	Co. B, 27th NCT
9	Hinnant, B. R.		
10	Hinson, John D. (3)	Stanly	Co. A, 57th NCT
11	Hinson, William H. (4)	Sampson, later Wayne	Co. H, 20th NCT
12	Hobbs, W. H. H.	Columbus	Co. H, 51st NCT
13	Hodgins, John M. (2) (also Hudgins)	Rowan	Co. D, 34th NCT (incorrectly listed as 54th NCT in Aud.)
14	Hoggard, James B.	Bertie	Co. G, 32nd NCT
15	Hoke, John D. (3) *(see also J. Pinckney Fry in CW Mil. 41)	Catawba	Co. K, 38th NCT

	Date	Limb	Location
1	22 Feb 1867 29 March 1867 (2)	Arm	Worth 4, letter Jewett Invoices Aud. 6.1, p. 25
2	19 April 1867	Arm	Aud. 6.1, p. 25
3	24 Feb 1866 22 Dec 1866 (2)	Leg	Worth 1, Co. List Jewett Invoices Aud. 6.1, p. 22
4	4 June 1867	Arm	Aud. 6.1, p. 26
5	28 Feb 1867	Arm	Aud. 6.1, p. 23
6	22 Sept 1866 6 Oct 1866 (2)	Leg	AG 58, p. 133 Jewett Invoices Aud. 6.1, p. 22
7	20 March 1866 7 Sept 1866 8 Sept 1866 (2)	Leg	Worth 2, Co. List AG 58, p. 113 Jewett Invoices Aud. 6.1, p. 22
8	no date 14 March 1867	Arm	Worth 8, City List Aud. 6.1, p. 23
9	6 April 1867		CW Military 41
10	24 Feb 1866 3 Oct 1866 (2)	Leg	Worth 1, Co. List Jewett Invoices Aud. 6.1, p. 22
11	15 Oct 1866 26 Nov 1866 (2) 27 Aug 1867	Leg	Worth 3, form Jewett Invoices Aud. 6.1, p. 23 CW Military 41
12	26 Feb 1867	Arm	Aud. 6.1, p. 26
13	12 July 1866 14 July 1866	Leg	Aud. 6.1, p. 23 Jewett Invoices
14	21 Nov 1883	Arm	CW Military 41
15	24 Feb 1866 16 April 1867 1 May 1867	Arm	Worth 1, Co. List CW Military 41* CW Mil, Co. List

	Claimant	County	Confederate Unit
1	Hoke, John W.	Catawba	Co. K, 38th NCT
2	Holden, J. W. (2)	Rowan	Co. F, 19th NCT (2nd NC Cav.)
3	Holleman, N. P.	Wake	Co. H, 3rd NCST
4	Holler, M. L.	Alexander	Co. K, 7th NCST
5	Hollowell, W. G. (3) (also Hallowell)	Wayne	Co. A, 27th NCT
6	Holt, A. (8) (Co. List includes an Archer Hol.)	Halifax	Co. G, 12th NCT
7	Holt, Robert A.	[Davie]	[Co. F, 13th NCT]
8	Holt, William	Alamance	
9	Holton, Thomas F. (3)	Mecklenburg	Co. K, 45th NCT
10	Honeycut, Bradford L. (5)	Iredell, McDowell, and Buncombe	Co. B, 19th NCT (2nd NC Cav.)
11	Honeycutt, Eli (2) (also Huneycutt)	Stanly	Co. C, 42nd NCT
12	Honeycutt, R. T. (2)	Cabarrus	Co. H, 8th NCST
13	Hooper, George	Halifax	
14	Hoover, Adolphus A. (2)	Catawba	Co. A, 12th NCT
15	Hopkins, M. F. (2)	Randolph	Co. H, 38th NCT

	Date	Limb	Location
1	25 April 1867	Arm	Aud. 6.1, p. 25
2	1 May 1867 27 May 1867	Arm	Worth 5, letter Aud. 6.1, p. 26
3	13 May 1867	Arm	Aud. 6.1, p. 25
4	12 March 1867	Arm	Aud. 6.1, p. 23
5	15 Jan 1867 16 Feb 1867 (2)	Leg	CW Military 41 Jewett Invoices Aud. 6.1, p. 24
6	5 March 1866 24 June 1866 Sept 1866 22 Sept 1866 26 Sept 1866 21 Feb 1867 24 Feb 1868 1 March 1868	Leg	Worth 2, Co. List Worth 3, form AG 58, p. 134 Aud. 6.1, p. 22 Jewett Invoices CW Military 41 Worth 8, letter PC 49.12, p. 331
7	19 June 1867		Worth 6, letter
8	10 March 1866	Leg	Worth 2, Co. List
9	14 Sept 1866 5 Jan 1867 7 Jan 1867	Leg	Worth 3, form Jewett Invoices Aud. 6.1, p. 22
10	3 April 1866 24 Jan 1867 1 July 1867 4 July 1867 (2)	Arm	Worth 2, Co. List CW Military 41 Aud. 6.1, p. 23 Worth 6, letter CW Military 41
11	24 Feb 1866 7 Feb 1867	Leg	Worth 1, Co. List Aud. 6.1, p. 24
12	22 June 1867 (2)	Arm	CW Military 41 Aud. 6.1, p. 25
13	5 March 1866	Arm	Worth 2, Co. List
14	24 Feb 1866 2 April 1867	Arm	Worth 1, Co. List Aud. 6.1, p. 24
15	30 Nov 1866 (2)	Leg	Jewett Invoices Aud. 6.1, p. 23

	Claimant	County	Confederate Unit
1	Hopson, J. A. (2)	Buncombe	Co. K, 25th NCT
2	Horney, W. A. (2) (also Harney)	Guilford	Co. B, 27th NCT
3	Horton, Fabius P. (4)	Wake	[Co. D], 8th NCST
4	Horton, Thomas J.	Rowan	Co. C, 41st NCT (3rd NC Cav.)
5	Houck, Washington	Ashe	[Co. A, 26th NCT]
6	Houk, Calvin	Burke	Home Guard
7	Houk, Michael	Ashe	Co. A, 26th NCT
8	House, B. A. (2)	Pitt	Co. B, 33rd NCT
9	Houser, Daniel (3)	Lincoln	Co. K, 49th NCT
10	Howard, Jonathan M. (4)	Union	Co. F, 49th NCT
11	Howell, M. B. (3)	Stanly	Co. C, 42nd NCT
12	Howell, P. C. (5)	Halifax	Co. G, 12th NCT
13	Howie, John N. (4)	Mecklenburg	Co. B, 53rd NCT

	Date	Limb	Location
1	10 May 1866 25 Feb 1867	Leg	Worth 2, Co. List Aud. 6.1, p. 23
2	27 Oct 1866 (2)	Leg	Jewett Invoices Aud. 6.1, p. 22
3	31 July 1866 23 March 1867 25 March 1867 no date	Leg	Worth 3, form CW Military 41 Aud. 6.1, p. 24 CW Mil, Co. List
4	27 April 1867	Arm	Aud. 6.1, p. 25
5	7 April 1866	Arm	Worth 2, Co. List
6	17 April 1867	Arm	Aud. 6.1, p. 25
7	27 Feb 1867	Arm	Aud. 6.1, p. 23
8	9 Oct 1866 (2)	Leg	Jewett Invoices Aud. 6.1, p. 22
9	11 Nov 1867 11 Dec 1867 (2)	Arm	CW Military 41 Aud. 6.1, p. 26 CW Military 41
10	22 Oct 1866 30 April 1867 4 May 1867 20 May 1867	Leg	Worth 3, Co. List CW Military 41 Aud. 6.1, p. 25 CW Military 41
11	24 Feb 1866 26 Feb 1867 (2)	Arm	Worth 1, Co. List CW Military 41 Aud. 6.1, p. 23
12	5 March 1866 29 Oct 1867 5 Dec 1867 7 Dec 1867 27 Dec 1867	Arm	Worth 2, Co. List CW Military 41 Aud. 6.1, p. 26 CW Military 41 CW Military 41
13	30 May 1866 6 Oct 1866 7 Dec 1866 (2)	Leg	Worth 2, form AG 58, p. 162 Jewett Invoices Aud. 6.1, p. 22

	Claimant	County	Confederate Unit
1	Hoyle, B. M. (2) (also Hoyl)	Cleveland	Co. F, 32nd NCT
2	Hoyle, Solomon (2)	Cleveland	Co. F, 55th NCT
3	Hoyler, Martin	Cleveland	
4	Hubbard, David A. (2)	Lincoln	Co. I, 11th NCT
5	Hubbard, James A.	Duplin	
6	Hubbard, James A. (3)	Forsyth	Co. A, 15th NCT
7	Hubbard, John N. (4)	Wake	Co. E, 14th NCT
8	Hudson, John W. (2)	Johnston	Co. E, 24th NCT
9	Hudson, Josiah (2)	Sampson	Co. H, 20th NCT
10	Huffman, Joel (2)	Alleghany	Co. A, 37th NCT
11	Huffstetler, John P. (3)	Gaston	Co. D, 37th NCT
12	Huggins, Augustus C., Sgt. Maj. (4)	Onslow	24th NCT
13	Hughes, James M. (3)	Alamance	Co. F, 54th NCT
14	Hughes, Peter	Alamance	Co. I, 8th NCST

15	Hughes, William (3)
	   (initials reported as W. H. H.
	   and W. M. H.)
		Cherokee	Co. A, 39th NCT

	Date	Limb	Location
1	no date 20 Nov 1866	Leg	Worth 8, Co. List Aud. 6.1, p. 22
2	27 Aug 1867 (2)	Arm	CW Military 41 Aud. 6.1, p. 25
3	16 Nov 1866	Leg	CW Military 41
4	May 1867 no date	Leg	Jewett Invoices Aud. 6.1, p. 24
5	13 Sept 1866	Leg	AG 58, p. 122
6	23 June 1866 18 Sept 1866 (2)	Leg	Worth 3, form Jewett Invoices Aud. 6.1, p. 22
7	13 June 1866 21 Aug 1866 (2) no date	Leg	Worth 3, form Jewett Invoices Aud. 6.1, p. 22 CW Mil, Co. List
8	5 March 1866 1 March 1867	Arm	Worth 2, Co. List Aud. 6.1, p. 23
9	25 June 1866 (2)	Leg	Jewett Invoices Aud. 6.1, p. 23
10	19 Nov 1867 (2)	Leg	Worth 7, form Aud. 6.1, p. 26
11	no date 22 Aug 1866 (2)	Leg	Worth 8, Co. List Jewett Invoices Aud. 6.1, p. 22
12	22 May 1866 15 Dec 1866 2 Feb 1867 (2)	Leg	CW Military 41 CW Military 41 Jewett Invoices Aud. 6.1, p. 24
13	27 Oct 1866 12 Dec 1866 (2)	Leg	Worth 3, form Jewett Invoices Aud. 6.1, p. 22
14	4 March 1867	Arm	Aud. 6.1, p. 23
15	20 July 1866 31 Oct 1866 (2)	Leg	Worth 3, form Jewett Invoices Aud. 6.1, p. 23

	Claimant	County	Confederate Unit
1	Humphry, William J. (4)	Robeson	Co. D, 51st NCT
2	Hunt, A. A. (2)	Franklin	Co. G, 47th NCT
3	Hunter, B. F. (2)	Wayne	Co. K, 19th Ga.
4	Hunter, J. W. (2)	Mecklenburg	[Co. C, 9th NCST (1st NC Cav.)]
5	Hunter, John V. (4) (also John P.)	Henderson and Buncombe	Co. F, 16th NCT
6	Hunter, John W. (2)	Davie	Co. F, 13th NCT
7	Hunter, Samuel (3)	Orange	Co. H, 56th NCT
8	Huntsinger, James	Polk	Co. A, 6th NCST
9	Hurley, W. P.		[Co. A, 26th NCT]
10	Hurst, Caswell (3) (also Hurse)	Wake	Co. H, 21st NCT [31st NCT in NCT *Roster*]
11	Hutchens, Silas	Orange	Co. C, 6th NCST
12	Hutcheson, John	Alamance	Co. H, 6th NCST
13	Hutchinson, John	Henderson	
14	Ingram, Hugh M. (3)	Anson	Co. H, 43rd NCT
15	Ireland, Robert L. (3)	Beaufort	Co. H, 7th Cavalry [Co. F, 16th Bn. NC Cav., in *NCT Roster*]
16	Irvin, John	Rockingham	[Co. G, 45th NCT]

	Date	Limb	Location
1	18 Oct 1867 (2) 26 Oct 1867 30 Oct 1867	Eyes	Worth 7, letters Aud. 6.1, p. 26 CW Military 41
2	1 March 1867 (2)	Leg	Jewett Invoices Aud. 6.1, p. 22
3	18 Feb 1867 (2)	Leg	Jewett Invoices Aud. 6.1, p. 24
4	9 Nov 1866 (2)	Foot	Worth 4, Co. List
5	16 April 1866 10 May 1866 10 June 1867 18 June 1867	Arm	Worth 2, Co. List Worth 2, Co. List CW Military 41 Aud. 6.1, p. 25
6	23 Nov 1867 (2)	Hand	CW Military 41 Aud. 6.1, p. 26
7	10 April 1867 25 April 1867 1 May 1867	Leg	Worth 5, letter Aud. 6.1, p. 25 CW Military 41
8	17 Aug 1867	Arm	Aud. 6.1, p. 25
9	25 Feb 1869	Arm	TC $ Bk 4, p. 201
10	21 Feb 1867 (2) no date	Arm	CW Military 41 Aud. 6.1, p. 23 CW Mil, Co. List
11	24 April 1867	Arm	Aud. 6.1, p. 25
12	12 March 1867	Arm	Aud. 6.1, p. 23
13	16 April 1866	Arm	Worth 2, Co. List
14	8 June 1866 8 Jan 1867 (2)	Leg	Worth 3, form Jewett Invoices Aud. 6.1, p. 27
15	26 Sept 1866 25 Feb 1867 (2)	Leg	Worth 3, form Jewett Invoices Aud. 6.1, p. 27
16	12 March 1866	Leg	CW Mil, Co. List

	Claimant	County	Confederate Unit
1	Isley, Peter (2) (also Iseley)	Alamance	Co. G, 44th NCT
2	Isley, Wesley (4) (also Iseley)	Alamance	Co. I, 57th NCT
3	Izzard, Sion (2)	Alamance	Co. B, 1st NCST
4	Jackson, John R.	Sampson	Co. I, 20th NCT
5	Jackson, Ollen M. (3) (erroneously given as Only Jackson in Co. List)	Harnett	[Co. B, 56th NCT]
6	Jacobs, Basil P. (2)	Macon	Co. K, 9th NCST (1st NC Cav.)
7	James, David H. (3) (listed as Davis H. James in Aud. and AG)	Pitt	Co. G, 8th NCST (incorrectly reported as 3rd NCT in Aud.)
8	James, Robinson	Sampson	Co. C, 51st NCT
9	Jarrett, G. W. (3)	Gaston	Co. H, 23rd NCT
10	Jarrett, J. M. (2)	Cleveland	Co. C, 15th NCT
11	Jenkins, Charles (2)	Bertie	Co.C, "Moore's Battalion" [3rd Bn. NC Light Arty.]
12	Jennings, George W. (3)	Mecklenburg	Co. K, 30th NCT
13	Jewell, James R. (3)	Craven	Co. B, 10th NCST (1st NC Arty.)
14	Jinnett, Joseph (2)	Wayne	Co. D, 67th NCT
15	Johnson, Charles L. (2)	Johnston	Co. A, 24th NCT

	Date	Limb	Location
1	26 Feb 1867 14 March 1867	Arm	CW Military 41 Aud. 6.1, p. 27
2	10 March 1866 27 Oct 1866 5 Dec 1866 (2)	Leg	Worth 2, Co. List Worth 3, form Jewett Invoices Aud. 6.1, p. 27
3	4 Sept 1867 (2)	Hand	CW Military 41 Aud. 6.1, p. 27
4	5 April 1867	Leg	Aud. 6.1, p. 27
5	5 Feb 1866 7 May 1867 2 June 1881	Leg and Arm	Worth 1, Co. List Aud. 6.1, p. 27 Aud. 6.1, p. 28
6	1 March 1867 23 Sept 1867	Leg	Worth 4, letter CW Military 41
7	24 Aug 1866 22 Sept 1866 (2)	Leg	AG 58, p. 97 Jewett Invoices Aud. 6.1, p. 27
8	22 April 1867	Leg	Aud. 6.1, p. 27
9	no date 15 Feb 1867 24 Aug 1867	Arm	Worth 8, Co. List CW Military 41 Aud. 6.1, p. 28
10	12 March 1867 16 March 1867	Leg	CW Military 41 Aud. 6.1, p. 28
11	27 Feb 1867 (2)	Arm	CW Military 41 Aud. 6.1, p. 27
12	23 July 1866 24 Aug 1866 (2)	Leg	Worth 3, form Jewett Invoices Aud. 6.1, p. 27
13	24 Aug 1866 11 Oct 1866 (2)	Leg	Worth 3, form Jewett Invoices Aud. 6.1, p. 27
14	20 March 1867 (2)	Leg	Jewett Invoices Aud. 6.1, p. 28
15	23 June 1868 24 June 1868	Arm	CW Military 41 Aud. 6.1, p. 28

	Claimant	County	Confederate Unit
1	Johnson, Edmund (2)	Cleveland	Co. E, 38th NCT
2	Johnson, George P. (4) (also Jonsthon and Johnston)	Wilkes	Co. B, 1st NCST
3	Johnson, James (4) (also Johnston)	Wilkes	Co. C, 26th NCT
4	Johnson, Matthew	Wake	Co. K, 42nd NCT
5	Johnson, Sylvester (2)	Wake	Co. H, 47th NCT
6	Johnson, W. S. (3)	New Hanover	Co. I, 20th NCT
7	Johnston, C. L.		
8	Johnston, Godfrey S. (2) (also Johnson)	Pitt	Co. H, 27th NCT
9	Johnston, J. G.	Mecklenburg	
10	Joines, S. F. (2) (also Joins)	Wilkes	[Co. D], 33rd NCT
11	Jones, Austin A. (3)	Wake	Co. G, 7th NCST
12	Jones, Grey (2)	Edgecombe	Co. I, 17th NCT (2nd organization)
13	Jones, Harper (3) (also Haper)	Guilford	Co. E, 22nd NCT
14	Jones, J. L. (2)	Wake	Co. D, 26th NCT
15	Jones, James A. (3)	Granville	Co. B, 12th NCT

	Date	Limb	Location
1	23 July 1867 (2)	Arm	CW Military 41 Aud. 6.1, p. 28
2	11 April 1866 1 Nov 1866 24 Oct 1867 2 Nov 1867	Arm	Worth 2, Co. List Worth 4, Co. List CW Military 41 Aud. 6.1, p. 28
3	11 April 1866 1 Nov 1866 23 Feb 1867 (2)	Arm	Worth 2, Co. List Worth 4, Co. List CW Military 41 Aud. 6.1, p. 28
4	[after 1868]	Leg	Aud. 6.1, p. 28
5	12 May 1867 15 May 1867	Leg	CW Military 41 Aud. 6.1, p. 27
6	5 Oct 1866 18 Oct 1866 (2)	Leg	AG 58, p. 152 Jewett Invoices Aud. 6.1, p. 27
7	24 June 1868	Arm	TC $ Bk 4, p. 95
8	16 Nov 1866 (2)	Leg	Jewett Invoices Aud. 6.1, p. 27
9	9 Nov 1866	Arm	Worth 4, Co. List
10	1 Nov 1866 21 Feb 1867	Arm	Worth 4, Co. List Aud. 6.1, p. 27
11	no date 12 Jun 1866 (2)	Leg	CW Mil, Co. List Aud. 6.1, p. 27 Jewett Invoices
12	29 Jan 1867 (2)	Leg	Jewett Invoices Aud. 6.1, p. 27
13	14 March 1867 no date (2)	Arm	Aud. 6.1, p. 28 Worth 8, Co. List and City List
14	21 May 1867 (2)	Knee	CW Military 41 Aud. 6.1, p. 27
15	12 March 1866 8 April 1867 28 May 1867	Arm	Worth 2, Co. List CW Military 41 Aud. 6.1, p. 28

	Claimant	County	Confederate Unit
1	Jones, John D. (4)	Forsyth	Co. K, 52nd NCT
2	Jones, Matthew	Davie	Co. G, 5th NCST
3	Jones, W. W. (2)	Jackson	[Co. G], Thomas's Legion
4	Jones, William R. (2)	Ashe	Co. A, 37th NCT
5	Jones, Zadock (2)	Onslow	[Co. B, 24th NCT]
6	Jordan, Thomas	Chowan	
7	Joyner, Isaac	Pitt	Co. G, 8th NCST
8	Joyner, J. C. (2)	Iredell	Co. H, 4th NCST
9	Justice, John G., Capt. (8)	Lincoln	"Hoke's Staff" [Hoke-Godwin-Lewis Brigade]
10	Justice, Theo. M. (4)	New Hanover	
11	Keener, David	Lincoln	[Co. H, 52nd NCT]
12	Keith, F. M. (2)	Wake	Co. C, 1st NCST
13	Keith, L. N. (2)	Wake	Co. K, 14th NCT
14	Kelly, D. P. (2)	Mecklenburg	Co. A, 33rd NCT

	Date	Limb	Location
1	8 March 1866 23 June 1866 27 July 1866 (2)	Leg	Worth 2, Co. List Worth 3, form Jewett Invoices Aud. 6.1, p. 27
2	20 March 1867	Arm	Aud. 6.1, p. 28
3	26 Feb 1867 (2)	Arm	CW Military 41 Aud. 6.1, p. 27
4	5 Jan 1869 9 Jan 1869	Leg	Aud 6.113 Aud 6.113
5	3 Dec 1866 23 Jan 1867	Leg	CW Military 41 Aud. 6.1, p. 27
6	27 Jan 1867	Arm	Aud. 6.1, p. 27
7	4 April 1867	Leg	Aud. 6.1, p. 27
8	3 April 1866 29 Aug 1867	Arm	Worth 2, Co. List Aud. 6.1, p. 28
9	16 July 1866 Sept 1866 6 Sept 1866 8 Oct 1866 18 Oct 1866 29 Oct 1866 30 Oct 1866 (2)	Leg	Worth 3, form CW Military 41 AG 58, p. 119 AG 58, p. 185 CW Military 41 CW Military 41 Jewett Invoices Aud. 6.1, p. 27
10	20 March 1867 1 April 1867 20 April 1867 25 May 1867	Arm	CW Military 41 Aud. 6.1, p. 28 CW Military 41 CW Military 41
11	17 June 1867		CW Military 41
12	8 June 1867 (2)	Leg	CW Military 41 Aud. 6.1, p. 29
13	6 June 1867 (2)	Arm	CW Military 41 Aud. 6.1, p. 29
14	21 March 1867 (2)	Arm	Worth 4, form Aud. 6.1, p. 29

	Claimant	County	Confederate Unit
1	Kelly, Henry H.	Bladen	Co. C, 1st Bn. NC Heavy Arty.
2	Kelly, J. J.	Wake	Co. C, 56th NCT
3	Kelly, James E.	Columbus	Co. E, 20th NCT (*NCT Roster* places Kelly in Co. K.)
4	Kelly, James H.	Orange	Co. I, 6th NCST
5	Kelly, Jefferson J.	Chatham	Co. F, 24th NCT
6	Kendall, Moses	Anson	Co. H, 43rd NCT
7	Kennedy, Robert (3)	Lenoir	Co. C, 27th NCT
8	Kernon, James M. (2) * (see also Bryan Buck in CW Mil. 41)	Beaufort	Co. I, 40th NCT
9	Kerr, John B. (4) (also Keer)	Alamance	Co. H, 57th NCT
10	Kersey, Clarkson L. (3) (given as C. N. on City List)	Guilford	Co. G, 22nd NCT
11	Kestler, William H.	Cabarrus	
12	Ketchum, John (3)	Onslow	Co. G, 3rd NCST
13	Kile, Henry (3)	McDowell	Co. D, 6th NCST
14	Kimbrough, J. T. (2)	Caswell	Co. A, 13th NCT
15	Kindrick, L. G.	Cleveland	Co. F, 34th NCT
16	King, (brother of Miles)	Warren	

	Date	Limb	Location
1	20 Dec 1867	Leg	Aud. 6.1, p. 30
2	9 April 1867	Arm	Aud. 6.1, p. 29
3	21 Feb 1867	Arm	Aud. 6.1, p. 29
4	5 Nov 1867	Arm	Aud. 6.1, p. 30
5	14 Feb 1868	Arm	Aud. 6.1, p. 30
6	25 April 1867	Arm	Aud. 6.1, p. 29
7	20 March 1866 13 Feb 1867 (2)	Leg	Worth 2, Co. List Jewett Invoices Aud. 6.1, p. 29
8	19 May 1867 28 May 1867	Arm	CW Military 41* Aud. 6.1, p. 29
9	10 March 1866 18 June 1866 1 Aug 1866 (2)	Leg	Worth 2, Co. List Worth 3, form Jewett Invoices Aud. 6.1, p. 29
10	1 May 1867 no date (2)	Arm	Aud. 6.1, p. 29 Worth 8, Co. List and City List
11	27 Feb 1867	Arm	CW Military 41
12	3 Dec 1866 8 Feb 1867 (2)	Leg	CW Military 41 Jewett Invoices Aud. 6.1, p. 29
13	31 May 1866 8 Jan 1867 (2)	Leg	Worth 2, Co. List Jewett Invoices Aud. 6.1, p. 29
14	21 June 1867 (2)	Leg	CW Military 41 Aud. 6.1, p. 29
15	8 April 1867	Arm	Aud. 6.1, p. 29
16	6 May 1868	Arm	CW Military 41

	Claimant	County	Confederate Unit
1	King, Allen (3)	Wayne	Co. A, 27th NCT
2	King, Calvin	Rockingham	
3	King, John E.	Rockingham	Co. F, 45th NCT
4	King, Richard M.	Warren	[Co. A, 14th NCT]
5	King, Thomas E. (3)	Halifax	Co. A, 14th NCT
6	King, Thomas E. (3)	New Hanover	2nd Co. I, 10th NCST (1st NC Arty.)
7	Kingsley, John H. (2)	Yadkin	
8	Kirkman, Julen A.	Guilford	
9	Kirkman, William	Mecklenburg	Co B, 2nd NCST
10	Kirtzel, H. L.	Catawba	
11	Kiser, David W.	Stanly	Co. I, 37th NCT
12	Kiser, E. H. (3) (also Kizer)	Forsyth	Co. I, 33rd NCT
13	Kiser, Marcus L. (3)	Cabarrus and Mecklenburg	Co. H, 57th NCT
14	Kisiah, Pinkney C. (3)	Mecklenburg	Co. F, 35th NCT
15	Kistler, Moses E. (2)	Mecklenburg	Co. F, 63rd NCT (5th NC Cav.)
16	Kistler, William H. (2)	Cabarrus	Co. B, 42nd NCT
17	Kizer, Lafayett	Cabarrus	

	Date	Limb	Location
1	24 March 1867 22 April 1867 (2)	Arm	CW Military 41 Jewett Invoices Aud. 6.1, p. 29
2	12 March 1866	Arm	CW Mil, Co. List
3	29 April 1867	Arm	Aud. 6.1, p. 29
4	11 March 1868		CW Military 41
5	11 May 1868 (3)	Arm	CW Military 41 TC $ Bk 4, p. 89 Aud. 6.1, p. 30
6	4 April 1867 5 April 1867 8 April 1867	Arm	CW Military 41 Aud. 6.1, p. 29 CW Military 41
7	15 Jan 1868 26 Feb 1868	Arm	CW Military 41 Aud. 6.1, p. 30
8	8 April 1867	Hand	CW Military 41
9	5 March 1868	Arm	Aud. 6.1, p. 30
10	12 June 1866	Leg	AG 58, p. 10
11	11 March 1867	Arm	Aud. 6.1, p. 29
12	11 April 1867 26 April 1867 8 May 1867	Leg	Worth 5, form Aud. 6.1, p. 29 CW Military 41
13	25 March 1867 27 March 1867 26 April 1867	Arm	CW Military 41 Aud. 6.1, p. 29 CW Military 41
14	3 July 1866 31 Oct 1866 (2)	Leg	Worth 3, form Jewett Invoices Aud. 6.1, p. 29
15	9 Nov 1866 25 March 1867	Arm	Worth 4, Co. List Aud. 6.1, p. 29
16	26 March 1866 2 March 1867	Arm	Worth 2, Co. List Aud. 6.1, p. 29
17	26 March 1866	Arm	Worth 2, Co. List

	Claimant	County	Confederate Unit
1	Knight, Benjamin (2)	Moore	Co. H, 30th NCT
2	Knipe, David		
3	Koonce, Henry C. (2)	Lenoir	Co. K, 61st NCT
4	Krider, C. C., Lt. (3)	Rowan	[Co. C], 49th NCT
5	Kriminger, E. J.	Union	[Co. A, 48th NCT]
6	Lackey, Dixon (5)	Cleveland and Gaston	Co. H, 34th NCT
7	Lackey, Wesley H. (2)	Alexander	Co. G, 38th NCT
8	Lambeth, A. M. (2) (erroneously listed as Lambert on invoice)	Randolph	Co. B, 23rd NCT
9	Lambeth, D. H. (2)	Davidson	Co. K, 27th NCT
10	Lamm, Thomas J. (3)	Wilson	Co. K, 66th NCT
11	Lancaster, L.		
12	Lancaster, Lawrence	Edgecombe	Co. F, 40th NCT
13	Lane, Thomas (2)	Stokes	Co. I, 33rd NCT
14	Lane, William (4)	Wilkes	[Co. E, 39th NCT]
15	Laney, Robert (2)	Caldwell	Co. I, 26th NCT

	Date	Limb	Location
1	6 Aug 1867 (2)	Hand	CW Military 41 Aud. 6.1, p. 30
2	17 May 1867	Arm	CW Military 41
3	15 Nov 1866 (2)	Leg	Jewett Invoices Aud. 6.1, p. 29
4	23 April 1866 7 Aug 1866 (2)	Leg	CW Mil, Co. List Jewett Invoices Aud. 6.1, p. 29
5	22 Oct 1866	Arm	Worth 3, Co. List
6	19 July 1867 24 July 1867 3 Aug 1867 10 Sept 1867 22 Sept 1867	Arm	Worth 6, letter Worth 6, letter Worth 6, letter CW Military 41 Aud. 6.1, p. 33
7	8 March 1867 12 March 1867	Arm	CW Military 41 Aud. 6.1, p. 32
8	21 Nov 1866 (2)	Leg	Aud. 6.1, p. 31 Jewett Invoices
9	15 May 1867 (2)	Arm	Jewett Invoices Aud. 6.1, p. 32
10	27 Dec 1866 1 Feb 1867 (2)	Leg	CW Military 41 Jewett Invoices Aud. 6.1, p. 31
11	7 March 1867	Leg	CW Military 41
12	13 March 1868	Arm	Aud. 6.1, p. 33
13	29 July 1867 30 Aug 1867	Leg	CW Military 41 Aud. 6.1, p. 32
14	11 April 1866 1 Nov 1866 23 Feb 1867 (2)	Arm	Worth 2, Co. List Worth 4, Co. List CW Military 41 Aud. 6.1, p. 33
15	18 Feb 1868 (2)	Hand	CW Military 41 Aud. 6.1, p. 33

	Claimant	County	Confederate Unit
1	Laney, Samuel L. (6)	Union	Co. B, 26th NCT
2	Langley, E. T.	Randolph	Co. M, 22nd NCT
3	Langley, James P. (4)	Onslow	Co. G, 3rd NCST
4	Langston, J. D. (4)	Wayne	Co. F, 10th NCST (1st NC Arty.)
5	Langston, William A. (3)	Johnston	Co. D, 5th NCST
6	Lassiter, T. B. (3) (also Lasater)	Chatham	Co. I, 32nd NCT
7	Latta, Willie P. (4)	Person	Co. A, 24th NCT
8	Lawrence, John (2)	Wake	Co. G, 1st NCST
9	Lawrence, William E. (4) (also Lowrance)	Catawba	Co. F, 3rd NCST
10	Lawson, Moses (3)	Stokes	Co. F, 21st NCT
11	Laxton, J. L. (3)	Burke	Co. F, 3rd NCST

	Date	Limb	Location
1	21 June 1866 7 Sept 1866 19 Sept 1866 (2) 21 May 1867 (2)	Leg	Worth 3, form AG 58, p. 114 Jewett Invoices Aud. 6.1, p. 31 CW Military 41
2	22 Nov 1867	Hand	Aud. 6.1, p. 33
3	3 Dec 1866 22 Feb 1867 26 Feb 1867 (2)	Leg	CW Military 41 CW Military 41 Jewett Invoices Aud. 6.1, p. 31
4	1 Aug 1866 16 Jan 1867 22 Feb 1867 (2)	Leg	Worth 3, form CW Military 41 Jewett Invoices Aud. 6.1, p. 31
5	5 March 1866 1 March 1867 (2)	Arm	Worth 2, Co. List CW Military 41 Aud. 6.1, p. 31
6	5 Dec 1866 2 March 1867 (2)	Arm	Worth 4, Co. List CW Military 41 Aud. 6.1, p. 31
7	26 May 1866 27 Nov 1866 24 Jan 1867 (2)	Leg	Worth 2, form Worth 4, Co. List Jewett Invoices Aud. 6.1, p. 31
8	no date 24 April 1867	Leg	CW Mil, Co. List Aud. 6.1, p. 31
9	24 Feb 1866 30 Nov 1866 26 Dec 1866 (2)	Leg	Worth 1, Co. List Worth 4, form Jewett Invoices Aud. 6.1, p. 31
10	2 Feb 1867 21 Feb 1867 (2)	Leg	CW Military 41 Jewett Invoices Aud. 6.1, p. 31
11	30 June 1866 25 July 1866 (2)	Leg	Worth 3, form Jewett Invoices Aud. 6.1, p. 31

	Claimant	County	Confederate Unit
1	Leary, James T. (3) (also Lurry)	Anson	Co. K, 43rd NCT
2	Ledford, Samuel E. (3)	Madison	[Co. C], 64th NCT
3	Lefler, Coleman (3)	Stanly	Co. D, 28th NCT
4	Lemons, P. D.	Rockingham	Co. G, 45th NCT
5	Lenoir, W. W. (3) (This is Capt. Walter W. Lenoir.)	Caldwell	Co. A, 37th NCT
6	Lenoir, W. W.	Haywood	
7	Leonard, Wiley (3) (also Willie)	Davidson	Co. B, 48th NCT
8	Leonard, William	Union	
9	Leonard, William J. (2)	Anson	Co. K, 43rd NCT
10	Leslie, J. O.	Rowan	Co. B, 2nd NC Cav.
11	Lewellin, Jackson	Rockingham	
12	Lewellin, R. J. (3)	Rockingham	Co. D, 45th NCT
13	Lewis, John I.	Edgecombe	Co. F, 30th NCT
14	Lillard, H. C.	Rockingham	Co. G, 45th NCT
15	Lilly, E. J. (2)	Montgomery	Co. C, 23rd NCT
16	Lindsay, M. H.	Orange	Co. F, 6th NCST
17	Lindsay, Wade (2)	Yadkin	Co. I, 18th NCT
18	Linebarger, David A. (2) (also Lineberger)	Gaston	Co. B, 28th NCT

	Date	Limb	Location
1	8 June 1866 19 Feb 1867 (2)	Leg	Worth 3, form Jewett Invoices Aud. 6.1, p. 31
2	10 March 1868 3 April 1868	Leg	CW Military 41 Aud. 6.1, p. 33
3	24 Feb 1866 22 Dec 1866 (2)	Leg	Worth 1, Co. List Jewett Invoices Aud. 6.1, p. 31
4	30 May 1867	Arm	Aud. 6.1, p. 32
5	27 June 1868 30 June 1868 (2)	Foot	CW Military 41 TC $ Bk 4, p. 95 Aud. 6.1, p. 33
6	15 May 1866	Leg	Worth 2, Co. List
7	31 May 1866 22 Nov 1866 (2)	Leg	Worth 2, form Jewett Invoices Aud. 6.1, p. 32
8	22 Oct 1866	Leg	Worth 3, Co. List
9	4 June 1867 17 Aug 1867	Leg	CW Military 41
10	19 March 1867	Arm	Aud. 6.1, p. 32
11	12 March 1866	Leg	CW Mil, Co. List
12	21 Aug 1866 8 Sept 1866 28 Sept 1866 (2)	Leg	Worth 3, form AG 58, p. 115 Jewett Invoices Aud. 6.1, p. 31
13	20 Dec 1867	Arm	Aud. 6.1, p. 33
14	6 May 1867	Arm	Aud. 6.1, p. 32
15	23 Jan 1867	Leg	Jewett Invoices Aud. 6.1, p. 31
16	9 April 1867	Arm	Aud. 6.1, p. 32
17	16 Jan 1867 26 Jan 1867	Leg	Worth 4, letter Aud. 6.1, p. 31
18	no date 27 Feb 1867	Arm	Worth 8, Co. List Aud. 6.1, p. 31

	Claimant	County	Confederate Unit
1	Linebarger, W. Alexander (3)	Catawba	Co. G, 12th NCT
2	Lineberger, E. F.	Gaston	[Co. M, 16th NCT]
3	Lingle, William A. (3)	Caldwell	Co. A, 22nd NCT
4	Linker, Jackson (3)	Cabarrus	[Co. B, 7th NCST]
5	Linker, William (2)	Cabarrus	Co. E, 59th NCT (4th NC Cav.)
6	Linnens, Samuel (4)	Alamance	Co. K, 47th NCT
7	Linster, McAfee (2)	Rowan	Co. E, 42nd NCT
8	Litaker, John A.	Cabarrus	Co. K, 57th NCT
9	Little, B. F., Col. (4)	Richmond	52nd NCT
10	Lockerman, John M.	Sampson	Co. C, 36th NCT
11	Loftin, Eli A. (2)	Rowan and Catawba	Co. F. 23rd NCT
12	Lofton, Anderson	Catawba	
13	Logan, L. C. (2)	Surry	Co. H, 21st NCT
14	Loggans, Naaman (2) (also Loggins)	Ashe	Co. A, 26th NCT
15	London, J. W. (2)	Burke	Co. B, 11th NCT
16	Long, Daniel (3)	Columbus	Co. D, 31st NCT

	Date	Limb	Location
1	24 Feb 1866 7 May 1867 11 May 1867	Arm	Worth 1, Co. List CW Military 41 Aud. 6.1, p. 32
2	no date	Arm	Worth 8, Co. List
3	7 July 1866 14 April 1868 (2)	Arm	CW Military 41 Aud. 6.1, p. 33 CW Military 41
4	26 March 1866 16 Feb 1867 (2)	Leg	Worth 2, Co. List CW Military 41 Aud. 6.1, p. 31
5	26 March 1866 16 Feb 1867	Leg	Worth 2, Co. List Aud. 6.1, p. 31
6	10 March 1866 27 Oct 1866 5 March 1867 (2)	Leg	Worth 2, Co. List Worth 3, letter Jewett Invoices Aud. 6.1, p. 31
7	26 March 1867 27 March 1867	Arm	CW Military 41 Aud. 6.1, p. 32
8	25 April 1867	Arm	Aud. 6.1, p. 32
9	11 April 1866 16 April 1867 3 June 1867 15 July 1867	Arm	Worth 2, Co. List CW Military 41 Aud. 6.1, p. 33 CW Military 41
10	11 April 1867	Arm	Aud. 6.1, p. 32
11	29 Jan 1867 30 Jan 1867	Leg	CW Military 41 Aud. 6.1, p. 31
12	24 Feb 1866	Leg	Worth 1, Co. List
13	18 Sept 1867 22 Feb 1868	Arm	Aud. 6.1, p. 32 CW Military 41
14	27 Feb 1867 14 July 1867	Leg	Aud. 6.1, p. 31 CW Military 41
15	25 March 1867 27 March 1867	Arm	CW Military 41 Aud. 6.1, p. 32
16	28 March 1867 2 April 1867 8 April 1867	Eyes	CW Military 41 Aud. 6.1, p. 32 CW Military 41

	Claimant	County	Confederate Unit
1	Long, George J.	Rowan and Alamance	Co. E, 1st NCST
2	Long, Rufus K. (3)	Rockingham	Co. D, 45th NCT
3	Long, William	Cleveland	Co. H, 34th NCT
4	Looper, O. H. (2)	Alexander	Co. G, 38th NCT
5	Loory, John	Rowan	Co. H, 14th NCT
6	Love, J. W. (2)	Caswell	Co. H, 24th NCT
7	Love, Jonah A. (2)	Stanly	Co. H, 42nd NCT
8	Low, C. A.	Burke	
9	Lowder, Daniel R.	Rowan	Co. D, 34th NCT
10	Lowder, G. W.	Stanly	Co. I, 52nd NCT
11	Lowder, W. P.	Stanly	Co. I, 52nd NCT
12	Lowrie, James A. (2) (also Lowery)	Guilford	Co. D, 57th NCT
13	Lowrie, John (4) (also Lowry)	Stanly	Co. H, 14th NCT (Leg returned in 1870 for $50 commutation.)
14	Lowry—see Loory		
15	Loy, Madison	Alamance	Co. K, 47th NCT
16	Lucas, Daniel	Harnett	Co. A, 10th Bn. NC Heavy Arty.
17	Lurry—see Leary		
18	Lyalls, William (2)	Ashe	Co. A, 34th NCT
19	Lynn, Thomas H. (3)	Cleveland	Co. F, 5th SC
20	Lytaker, T. A.	Cabarrus	

	Date	Limb	Location
1	1 April 1867	Fingers	CW Military 41
2	18 May 1868 (3)	Leg	Worth 8, letter TC $ Bk 4, p. 91 Aud. 6.1, p. 31
3	8 April 1867	Arm	Aud. 6.1, p. 32
4	17 Dec 1867 (2)	Hand	CW Military 41 Aud. 6.1, p. 33
5	19 Dec 1882	Leg	CW Military 41
6	15 June 1867 25 June 1867	Arm	CW Military 41 Aud. 6.1, p. 32
7	24 Feb 1866 11 April 1867	Arm	Worth 1, Co. List Aud. 6.1, p. 32
8	10 Aug 1866	Leg	AG 58, p. 70
9	12 March 1867	Arm	Aud. 6.1, p. 32
10	29 May 1867	Arm	Aud. 6.1, p. 32
11	29 May 1867	Arm	Aud. 6.1, p. 32
12	no date 6 Sept 1866	Arm	Worth 8, City List Aud. 6.1, p. 33
13	24 Feb 1866 16 Jan 1867 (2) 6 April 1870	Leg	Worth 1, Co. List Jewett Invoices Aud. 6.1, p. 31 Aud. 6.1, p. 67
14			
15	4 March 1867	Arm	Aud. 6.1, p. 32
16	13 May 1867	Arm	Aud. 6.1, p. 32
17			
18	7 April 1866 30 April 1867	Arm	Worth 2, Co. List Aud. 6.1, p. 32
19	no date 12 March 1867 16 March 1867	Arm	Worth 8, Co. List CW Military 41 Aud. 6.1, p. 32
20	26 March 1866	Arm	Worth 2, Co. List

	Claimant	County	Confederate Unit
1	Mabry, Joseph (2)	Stanly	Co. H, 14th NCT
2	Mace, Jesse (4)	Mitchell	Co. A, 58th NCT
3	Mahler, J. M.	Wilkes	Co. B, 55th NCT
4	Mall, Irwin		
5	Mallard, William W. (4)	Duplin	Co. E, 30th NCT
6	Malloch, Atlas F. (3) (also Maloch and Malock)	Richmond	Co. D, 23rd NCT
7	Malone, Nathaniel (5)	Alamance	Co. K, 6th NCT
8	Malpass, Lewis Frank	Lenoir	[Co. E, 61st NCT]
9	Malpass, Lewis Henry (3)	New Hanover	Co. E, 18th NCT
10	Mangum, P. G. (2)	Wake	Co. E, 47th NCT
11	Mangum, Theophilus P. (2)	Wake	Co. D, 30th NCT
12	Manly, J. A.	Stokes	Co. F, 45th NCT
13	Manning, James (2)	Mecklenburg	Co. I, 37th NCT
14	Manuel, Hugh (5)	Rockingham	Co. H, 22nd NCT

	Date	Limb	Location
1	22 June 1867 (2)	Hand	CW Military 41 Aud. 6.1, p. 38
2	5 April 1867 11 April 1867 26 April 1867 30 April 1867	Arm	CW Military 41 Aud. 6.1, p. 37 CW Military 41 CW Military 41
3	10 Oct 1867	Arm	Aud. 6.1, p. 38
4	1 April 1867		CW Military 41
5	19 April 1866 4 Dec 1866 (2) 1 Nov 1867	Leg	CW Mil, Co. List Jewett Invoices Aud. 6.1, p. 34 Worth 7, letter
6	11 April 1866 19 Dec 1866 (2)	Leg	Worth 2, Co. List Jewett Invoices Aud. 6.1, p. 35
7	10 March 1866 27 Oct 1866 14 Nov 1866 27 Nov 1866 (2)	Leg	Worth 2, Co. List Worth 3, letter CW Military 41 Jewett Invoices Aud. 6.1, p. 35
8	20 March 1866	Arm	Worth 2, Co. List
9	22 April 1867 25 April 1867 6 May 1867	Hand	CW Military 41 Aud. 6.1, p. 37 CW Military 41
10	30 May 1867 31 May 1867	Leg	Aud. 6.1, p. 38 CW Military 41
11	3 June 1867 24 June 1867	Arm	CW Military 41 Aud. 6.1, p. 38
12	13 March 1867	Arm	Aud. 6.1, p. 36
13	27 March 1867 30 March 1867	Arm	CW Military 41 Aud. 6.1, p. 33
14	12 March 1866 27 Aug 1866 28 Aug 1866 26 Oct 1866 27 Oct 1866	Leg	CW Mil, Co. List Worth 3, form Worth 3, letter Aud. 6.1, p. 34 Jewett Invoices

	Claimant	County	Confederate Unit
1	Marlow, Martin (2)	Wilkes	[Co. B, 55th NCT]
2	Maron, Sam	Chatham	
3	Marsh, John W. (2) *(see also Elkanah Cloninger in CW Mil. 41)	Catawba	Co. B, 32nd NCT
4	Marsh, Thomas A.	Guilford	Co. B, 6th NCST
5	Marsh, Wesley	Catawba	
6	Marshburn, James N. (2) (also Mashburn)	New Hanover	Co. H, 11th NCT
7	Martin, George (3)	Gaston	Co. C, 38th NCT
8	Martin, Jeremiah	Stokes	Co. E, 7th NC Reserves
9	Martin, Lewis (4)	Wayne	Co. I, 16th NCT
10	Martin, Thomas P. (2)	Polk	Co. I, 5th NCST
11	Mashburn, H. R. (2) (also H. B. Marshburn)	Duplin	Co. B, 3rd NCST
12	Massey, Rufus	Orange	Co. C, 5th NCST
13	Mast, D. P. (4)	Caldwell	Co. D, 9th NCST (1st NC Cav.)
14	Matheson, D. Mc.	Alexander	[Co. G, 38th NCT]
15	Mathis, Noel (3) (also Matthis)	Wilson	Co. K, 66th NCT
16	Matthews, Benjamin W. (3)	Harnett	Co. E, 47th NCT

	Date	Limb	Location
1	11 April 1866 1 Nov 1866	Arm	Worth 2, Co. List Worth 4, Co. List
2	5 Dec 1866	Leg	Worth 4, Co. List
3	22 March 1867 2 April 1867	Arm	CW Military 41* Aud. 6.1, p. 36
4	25 March 1867	Leg	Aud. 6.1, p. 35
5	24 Feb 1866	Arm	Worth 1, Co. List
6	1 Feb 1867 (2)	Leg	Jewett Invoices Aud. 6.1, p. 34
7	no date 21 Sept 1866 (2)	Leg	Worth 8, Co. List Jewett Invoices Aud. 6.1, p. 34
8	2 April 1867	Arm	Aud. 6.1, p. 36
9	21 Feb 1868 28 Feb 1868 1 March 1868 7 March 1868	Arm	CW Military 41 Aud. 6.1, p. 33 CW Military 41 CW Military 41
10	17 April 1866 6 May 1867	Arm	Worth 2, Co. List Aud. 6.1, p. 37
11	14 Jan 1867 (2)	Arm	Jewett Invoices Aud. 6.1, p. 35
12	23 April 1867	Arm	Aud. 6.1, p. 37
13	7 July 1866 16 Oct 1866 19 Nov 1866 (2)	Leg	Worth 3, form Worth 3, letter Jewett Invoices Aud. 6.1, p. 35
14	12 March 1867	Arm	Aud. 6.1, p. 36
15	5 Aug 1867 8 Aug 1867 13 Aug 1867	Arm	CW Military 41 Aud. 6.1, p. 38 CW Military 41
16	5 Feb 1866 12 March 1867 15 March 1867	Arm	Worth 1, Co. List CW Military 41 Aud. 6.1, p. 36

	Claimant	County	Confederate Unit
1	Matthews, Daniel (2)	Cumberland	[Co. C, 36th NCT (2nd NC Arty.)]
2	Matthews, James (3)	Granville	Co. A, 44th NCT
3	Matthews, Thomas (2)	Bertie	
4	Matthis, W. A.	Sampson	Co. A, 63rd NCT (5th NC Cav.)
5	Maxwell, Robert	Mecklenburg	[Co. C, 9th NCST (1st NC Cav.)]
6	Mayhew, William Newton (2)	Rowan	Co. B, 46th NCT
7	Maynard, James P. (4)	Granville	Co. G, 23rd NCT
8	Maze, A. F.	Stokes	Co. A, 2nd Bn. Arty.
9	McAdams, J. F.	Orange	Co. F, 33rd NCT
10	McAlphin, J. J.	Duplin	Co. I, 1st NCT
11	McArthur, N. J.	Sampson	Co. F, 20th NCT
12	McBryde, Duncan ("disabled")	Robeson	[Co. G, 24th NCT]
13	McCaddin, William W. (2)	Davidson	Co. D, 24th NCT
14	McCall, John A. (2)	Mecklenburg	Co. I, 48th NCT
15	McCrodan, Robert (2)	Warren	[Co. K, 12th NCT]
16	McCrory, Julius S. (2)	Person	Co. A, 24th NCT

	Date	Limb	Location
1	21 March 1867 23 March 1867	Hand	CW Military 41 Aud. 6.1, p. 36
2	12 March 1866 17 April 1867 28 May 1867	Arm	Worth 2, Co. List CW Military 41 Aud. 6.1, p. 37
3	27 Feb 1867 (2)	Arm	CW Military 41 Aud. 6.1, p. 35
4	22 April 1867	Arm	Aud. 6.1, p. 37
5	9 Nov 1866	Arm	Worth 4, Co. List
6	23 April 1866 15 March 1867	Arm	CW Mil, Co. List Aud. 6.1, p. 36
7	12 March 1866 14 June 1866 21 July 1866 (2)	Leg	Worth 2, Co. List Worth 3, form Jewett Invoices Aud. 6.1, p. 34
8	1 July 1867	Arm	Aud. 6.1, p. 36
9	9 April 1867	Arm	Aud. 6.1, p. 36
10	2 April 1867	Arm	Aud. 6.1, p. 36
11	22 April 1867	Arm	Aud. 6.1, p. 36
12	10 Oct 1866		Worth 3, Co. List
13	9 March 1868 16 March 1868	Arm	CW Military 41 Aud. 6.1, p. 33
14	9 July 1867 9 Aug 1867	Leg	CW Military 41 Aud. 6.1, p. 38
15	1 Feb 1868 8 Feb 1868	Arm	CW Military 41 Aud. 6.1, p. 33
16	27 Nov 1866 9 March 1867	Arm	Worth 4, Co. List Aud. 6.1, p. 35

	Claimant	County	Confederate Unit
1	McCrory, William (5) (also McRorie)	Union	Co. B, 26th NCT
2	McCuistin, James (2) (also McCuiston)	Guilford	Co. A, 34th NCT
3	McDade, John	Wake	Co. E, 47th NCT
4	McDade, William P. (2)	Orange	Co. E, 31st NCT
5	McDaniel, Christopher (2)	Burke	Co. E, 6th NCT (Co. C in *NCT Roster*)
6	McDaniel, Franklin H. (3) (One Co. List includes an L. H.)	Wilkes	Co. C, 26th NCT
7	McDaniel, John	Jones	Co. G, 2nd NCST
8	McGalliard, James W. (2)	Burke	Co. E, 16th NCT
9	McGin, Isaac H.	Mecklenburg	[Co. B, 13th NCT]
10	McGin, James	Mecklenburg	
11	McGin, W. A.	Mecklenburg	[Co. B, 13th NCT]
12	McGinn, J. H. (4)	Mecklenburg	Co. B, 13th NCT
13	McKee, H. A.	Orange	Co. E, 31st NCT
14	McLain, J. F.	Alexander	Co. E, 37th NCT
15	McLauchlin, A. H. (5)	Robeson	Co. G, 24th NCT
16	McLauchlin, B. J.	Robeson	

	Date	Limb	Location
1	30 June 1866 6 Aug 1866 15 Sept 1866 3 Nov 1866 (2)	Leg	Worth 3, form Worth 3, letter CW Military 41 Jewett Invoices Aud. 6.1, p. 34
2	no date 14 March 1867	Arm	Worth 8, City List Aud. 6.1, p. 36
3	4 May 1867	Arm	Aud. 6.1, p. 37
4	24 April 1867 27 April 1867	Arm	Worth 5, letter Aud. 6.1, p. 37
5	20 April 1867 24 April 1867	Leg	Worth 5, letter Aud. 6.1, p. 37
6	11 April 1866 1 Nov 1866 29 March 1867	Leg	Worth 2, Co. List Worth 4, Co. List Aud. 6.1, p. 33
7	20 Dec 1867	Eyes	Aud. 6.1, p. 33
8	2 May 1867 13 May 1867	Arm	Aud. 6.1, p. 37 CW Military 41
9	9 Nov 1866	Foot	Worth 4, Co. List
10	9 Nov 1866	Leg	Worth 4, Co. List
11	9 Nov 1866	Foot	Worth 4, Co. List
12	30 May 1866 23 July 1866 (3)	Foot	Worth 2, form Jewett Invoices CW Military 41 Aud. 6.1, p. 34
13	27 March 1867	Arm	Aud. 6.1, p. 36
14	12 March 1867	Arm	Aud. 6.1, p. 35
15	3 July 1866 20 Aug 1866 5 Oct 1866 28 Nov 1866 (2)	Leg	Worth 3, form Worth 3, letter AG 58, p. 147 Jewett Invoices Aud. 6.1, p. 34
16	10 Oct 1866	Leg	Worth 3, Co. List

	Claimant	County	Confederate Unit
1	McLauchlin, John M.	Richmond	[Co. H, 36th NCT (2nd NC Arty.)]
2	McLean, Abner	Mecklenburg	Co. D, 7th NCST
3	McLean, David	Wilkes	Co. B, 1st NCST
4	McLean, Joseph M. (4)	Guilford	Co. M, 21st NCT
5	McLeod, Samuel	Caldwell	Co. H, 58th NCT
6	McLure, Joseph A. (2)	Mecklenburg	Co. K, 30th NCT
7	McMatheson, D.	Alexander	
8	McMillan, Roderick	Robeson	[Co. K, 38th NCT]
9	McNairy, John W. (5)	Guilford and Randolph	Co. B, 27th NCT
10	McNeely, Jonathan	Cleveland	Co. F, 55th NCT
11	McNeely, Thomas Henry (3) (erroneously listed as J. H. in Aud.)	Burke	Co. D, 6th NCST
12	McNeill, A. E. (5)	Robeson	Co. G, 24th NCT
13	McNeill, Hector M. (3)	Harnett	Co. E, 56th NCT
14	McNeill, Jesse H. (3) (also McNiel)	Wilkes	Co. K, 53rd NCT
15	McNeill, Lauchlin	Moore	Co. H, 30th NCT

	Date	Limb	Location
1	14 July 1867	Hand	Worth 6, letter
2	10 May 1867	Arm	Aud. 6.1, p. 37
3	14 Sept 1867	Arm	Aud. 6.1, p. 38
4	23 Feb 1867 11 March 1867 no date (2)	Arm	CW Military 41 Aud. 6.1, p. 35 Worth 8, Co. List and City List
5	26 April 1867	Arm	Aud. 6.1, p. 37
6	22 May 1868 (2)	Arm	TC $ Bk 4, p. 91 Aud. 6.1, p. 35
7	11 March 1867	Arm	CW Military 41
8	10 Oct 1866	Arm	Worth 3, Co. List
9	29 Oct 1866 1 Nov 1866 12 Dec 1866 (2) 26 Aug 1869	Leg	Worth 3, letter AG 58, p. 187 Jewett Invoices Aud. 6.1, p. 35 TC $ Bk 4, p. 271
10	15 Aug 1867	Arm	Aud. 6.1, p. 38
11	30 June 1866 23 Oct 1866 (2)	Leg	Worth 3, form Jewett Invoices Aud. 6.1, p. 34
12	21 Feb 1866 13 Dec 1867 1 Feb 1868 5 Feb 1868 2 March 1868	Hand	Worth 1 Co. List CW Military 41 Aud. 6.1, p. 33 CW Military 41 CW Military 41
13	5 Feb 1866 29 June 1866 (2)	Leg	Worth 1, Co. List Jewett Invoices Aud. 6.1, p. 34
14	11 April 1866 23 Feb 1867 (2)	Arm	Worth 2, Co. List CW Military 41 Aud. 6.1, p. 33
15	19 May 1867	Arm	Aud. 6.1, p. 37

	Claimant	County	Confederate Unit
1	McPhail, Dougald (3)	Harnett	Co. H, 50th NCT
2	McQuage, Alexander	Montgomery	Co. I, 43rd NCT
3	McRae, George A. (2)	Moore	Co. G, 63rd NCT (5th NC Cav.)
4	McSwain, William R. (2)	Stanly	Co. H, 2nd NCST
5	Meadows, John G. (3)	Granville	Co. D, 12th NCT
6	Mercer, Jacob I.	Edgecombe	Co. F, 30th NCT
7	Mercer, Miles V. (5)	Robeson	Co. B, 51st NCT
8	Merrit, Benjamin (3)	Halifax	Co. F, 35th Heavy Artillery [36th NCT (2nd NC Arty.) in NCT *Roster*]
9	Merrit, Marshal (3) (also Martial Merrit)	Bladen	Co. F, 36th NCT
10	Merritt, F. M. (2)	Sampson	Co. B, 51st NCT
11	Merritt, George H. (2)	Granville	Co. K, 44th NCT
12	Merry, Thomas (2) (Middle initial listed as both H. and O.)	Beaufort	[Co. E, 4th NCST]
13	Messer, F. M. (4)	Haywood	Co. C, 25th NCT

	Date	Limb	Location
1	5 Feb 1866 15 May 1867 (2)	Arm	Worth 1, Co. List CW Military 41 Aud. 6.1, p. 37
2	31 July 1867	Arm	Aud. 6.1, p. 38
3	18 Aug 1866 (2)	Leg	Jewett Invoices Aud. 6.1, p. 34
4	24 Feb 1866 16 April 1867	Arm	Worth 1, Co. List Aud. 6.1, p. 37
5	12 March 1866 16 April 1867 28 May 1867	Arm	Worth 2, Co. List CW Military 41 Aud. 6.1, p. 38
6	29 Nov 1867	Arm	Aud. 6.1, p. 33
7	21 Feb 1866 10 Oct 1866 9 Sept 1867 27 Sept 1867 5 Oct 1867	Arm	Worth 1, Co. List Worth 3, Co. List CW Military 41 CW Military 41 Aud. 6.1, p. 38
8	13 April 1868 16 April 1868 5 May 1868	Arm	CW Military 41 TC $ Bk 4, p. 89 Aud. 6.1, p. 62
9	10 April 1866 26 Feb 1867 (2)	Arm	Worth 2, Co. List CW Military 41 Aud. 6.1, p. 35
10	4 June 1867 (2)	Arm	CW Military 41 Aud. 6.1, p. 38
11	24 Oct 1867 (2)	Hand	CW Military 41 Aud. 6.1, p. 38
12	15 May 1866 3 Sept 1866	Leg	CW Military 41 Worth 3, form
13	15 May 1866 2 Feb 1867 31 Aug 1867 5 Oct 1867	Leg	Worth 2, Co. List CW Military 41 Worth 6, letter Aud. 6.1, p. 38

	Claimant	County	Confederate Unit
1	Mickey, T. E.	Stokes	Co. I, 33rd NCT
2	Miller, Jesse (2)	Rowan	Co. K, 5th NCST
3	Miller, John	Davidson	Co. I, 42nd NCT
4	Miller, L. F.	Davidson	Co. A, 48th NCT
5	Miller, Robert M. (5)	Rockingham	Co. G, 14th NCT
6	Miller, William P.	Rockingham	Co. E, 45th NCT
7	Mills, Bryan (2)	Onslow	Co. A, 35th NCT (erroneously reported as Co. H in Aud.)
8	Mills, John (2)	Pitt	Co. E, 55th NCT
9	Mills, T. D. (2)	Wilkes	Co. B, 26th NCT
10	Mills, W. F. (2)	Pitt	Co. I, [1st Bn. NC Local Defense Troops]
11	Mills, W. J. (2)	Wake	Co. D, 26th NCT
12	Millsaps, F. M. (2)	Jackson	Co. K, 39th NCT
13	Mince, T. J.	Rutherford	Co. I, 34th NCT
14	Mints, William D. (2)	Rutherford	Co. C, 5th Ark.
15	Mintz, William W. (3)	New Hanover	1st Co A, 36th NCT (2nd NC Arty.)
16	Mitchell, F. M. (3)	Alleghany	Co. I, 61st NCT (leg returned for $50 commutation in 1870)

	Date	Limb	Location
1	30 April 1867	Arm	Aud. 6.1, p. 37
2	23 April 1866 19 March 1867	Arm	CW Mil, Co. List Aud. 6.1, p. 33
3	9 April 1867	Arm	Aud. 6.1, p. 36
4	14 March 1867	Arm	Aud. 6.1, p. 36
5	2 Aug 1866 29 Aug 1866 27 Oct 1866 (2) 26 March 1867	Leg	Worth 3, form AG 58, p. 150 Jewett Invoices Aud. 6.1, p. 34 CW Military 41
6	13 May 1867	Arm	Aud. 6.1, p. 37
7	24 April 1867 13 May 1867	Arm	CW Military 41 Aud. 6.1, p. 37
8	25 Feb 1867 (2)	Arm	CW Military 41 Aud. 6.1, p. 35
9	20 Aug 1867 (2)	Arm	CW Military 41 Aud. 6.1, p. 38
10	25 Feb 1867 (2)	Arm	CW Military 41 Aud. 6.1, p. 35
11	23 May 1867 24 May 1867	Leg	CW Military 41 Aud. 6.1, p. 38
12	26 Feb. 1867 (2)	Arm	CW Military 41 Aud. 6.1, p. 35
13	1 July 1867	Arm	Aud. 6.1, p. 38
14	7 May 1867 (2)	Eyes	CW Military 41 Aud. 6.1, p. 33
15	20 April 1867 25 April 1867 4 May 1867	Arm	CW Military 41 Aud. 6.1, p. 37 CW Military 41
16	21 Feb 1866 (2) 25 Jan 1870	Leg	Jewett Invoices Aud. 6.1, p. 34 Aud. 6.1, p. 34

	Claimant	County	Confederate Unit
1	Mitchell, J. W. (2)	Alamance	Co. A, 27th NCT
2	Mitchell, Michael (3)	Watauga	Co. I, 58th NCT
3	Mitchell, Stephen R. (2)	Alamance	Co. K, 47th NCT
4	Mock, James A. (4)	Watauga	Co. F, 52nd NCT
5	Money, Daniel W. (2)	Yadkin	Co. H, 4th NCST
6	Montgomery, G. W. (2)	Montgomery	Co. F, 44th NCT
7	Montgomery, William P. (3)	Hertford	Co. F, 1st NCST
8	Moody, Hiram (2)	Burke	Co. K, 35th NCT
9	Moody, William J. (5)	Gates	Co. B, 5th NCST
10	Moon, Jackson (2)	Bertie	
11	Mooney, E. D.	Rutherford	Co. I, 56th NCT
12	Mooney, William (3)	Caldwell and Wilkes	Co. B, 1st NCST
13	Moore, David J. (2)	New Hanover	Co. E, 18th NCT

	Date	Limb	Location
1	19 March 1867 20 March 1867	Arm	CW Military 41 Aud. 6.1, p. 36
2	4 Sept 1866 30 Oct 1866 (2)	Leg	Worth 3, form Jewett Invoices Aud. 6.1, p. 34
3	2 April 1867 3 April 1867	Leg	CW Military 41 Aud. 6.1, p. 36
4	4 Sept 1866 8 Sept 1866 6 Oct 1866 (2)	Foot	Worth 3, form Worth 3, letter Jewett Invoices Aud. 6.1, p. 34
5	17 March 1867 26 March 1867	Arm	CW Military 41 Aud. 6.1, p. 35
6	2 May 1867 22 May 1867	Leg	CW Military 41 Aud. 6.1, p. 38
7	29 Dec 1866 15 Jan 1867 (2)	Leg	CW Military 41 Jewett Invoices Aud. 6.1, p. 34
8	1 May 1867 7 May 1867	Arm	CW Military 41 Aud. 6.1, p. 37
9	22 Aug 1866 27 Aug 1866 5 Oct 1866 28 Nov 1866 (2)	Leg	Worth 3, form Worth 3, letter AG 58, p. 150 Jewett Invoices Aud. 6.1, p. 34
10	27 Feb 1867 (2)	Arm	CW Military 41 Aud. 6.1, p. 35
11	30 May 1867	Arm	Aud. 6.1, p. 38
12	1 Nov 1866 17 Dec 1867 (2)	Arm	Worth 4, Co. List CW Military 41 Aud. 6.1, p. 33
13	2 March 1867 (2)	Eyes	CW Military 41 Aud. 6.1, p. 35

	Claimant	County	Confederate Unit
1	Moore, G. M. (2)	Cleveland	Co. H, 28th NCT
2	Moore, J. R. (3)	Burke	Co. K, 33rd NCT
3	Moore, Lewis (2)	Sampson	Co. C, 1st NCST
4	Moore, Luther (2)	Caldwell	Co. H, 58th NCT
5	Moore, W. H. H. (2)	Wake	Co. D, 30th NCT
6	Moore, William P. (2)	Person	Co. H, 24th NCT
7	Moore, William R. B. (4)	Washington	Co. G, 1st NC Cav.
8	Moorefield, Henderson	Stokes	Co. G, 53rd NCT
9	Mooring, William (2)	Greene	Co. K, 33rd NCT
10	Moose, John H. (3)	Cabarrus	Co. H, 8th NCST
11	Moran, Samuel	Alamance	Co. G, 26th NCT
12	Morgan, A. A. (2)	Burke	Co. B, 11th NCT
13	Morgan, Calvin (3)	Rowan	Co. G, 6th NCST
14	Morgan, Ivy C. (2)	Rowan	Co. K, 8th NCST
15	Morgan, Marshall H. (3)	New Hanover	Co. C, 1st NCST

	Date	Limb	Location
1	4 April 1867 8 April 1867	Leg	CW Military 41 Aud. 6.1, p. 36
2	30 June 1866 25 July 1866 (2)	Leg	Worth 3, form Jewett Invoices Aud. 6.1, p. 34
3	24 July 1867 24 Aug 1867	Leg	CW Military 41 Aud. 6.1, p. 38
4	5 June 1867 8 June 1867	Arm	CW Military 41 Aud. 6.1, p. 38
5	5 June 1867 6 June 1867	Arm	CW Military 41 Aud. 6.1, p. 38
6	27 Nov 1866 29 March 1867	Arm	Worth 4, Co. List Aud. 6.1, p. 36
7	15 Sept 1866 17 Oct 1866 25 Oct 1866 19 Nov 1866	Leg	Worth 3, form Worth 3, letter Jewett Invoices Aud. 6.1, p. 35
8	25 March 1867	Arm	Aud. 6.1, p. 36
9	21 Feb 1866 27 April 1867	Arm	Worth 1, Co. List Aud. 6.1, p. 37
10	26 March 1866 30 Jan 1867 27 March 1867	Arm	Worth 2, Co. List CW Military 41 Aud. 6.1, p. 35
11	29 April 1867	Leg	Aud. 6.1, p. 37
12	18 March 1867 25 March 1867	Arm	CW Military 41 Aud. 6.1, p. 36
13	23 April 1866 3 July 1866 (2)	Leg	CW Mil, Co. List Jewett Invoices Aud. 6.1, p. 34
14	1 April 1867 3 April 1867	Leg	CW Military 41 Aud. 6.1, p. 36
15	9 April 1867 11 April 1867 22 April 1867	Arm	CW Military 41 Aud. 6.1, p. 36 CW Military 41

	Claimant	County	Confederate Unit
1	Morgan, Solomon (2)	Rowan	Co. K, 57th NCT
2	Moring, James H. (2)	Orange	Co. I, 6th NCST
3	Morris, James	Halifax	[Co. F, 43rd NCT]
4	Morris, James S. (2)	Mecklenburg	Co. C, 10th NCST (1st NC Arty.)
5	Morris, Stephen W. (2)	Johnston	Co. G, 55th NCT
6	Morris, Z. W.	Buncombe	Co. K, 11th NCT
7	Morrison, J. G., Capt. (3)	Lincoln	Co. F, 57th NCT, and "General Jackson's Staff"
8	Morrison, L. M. (2)	Cabarrus	Co. H, 7th NCST
9	Morrison, McKee	Cabarrus	
10	Morrison, Rufus A. (3)	Iredell	Co. A, 7th NCST
11	Morriss, James H. (2)	Halifax	Co. F, 43rd NCT
12	Moser, Calvin	Catawba	
13	Moses, Luther H. (2)	Franklin	Co K, 12th NCT
14	Moss, James (2)	Cleveland	Co. C, 55th NCT
15	Motley, John R. (4)	Cabarrus	Co. B, 7th NCST
16	Mott, Daniel W. (3)	New Hanover	Co. D, 13th Bn. NC Light Arty.
17	Mullican, [Lewis] S.	Davie	[Co. G, 4th NCST]

	Date	Limb	Location
1	23 April 1866 15 March 1867	Arm	CW Mil, Co. List Aud. 6.1, p. 36
2	18 May 1867 20 May 1867	Leg	Worth 5, letter Aud. 6.1, p. 38
3	5 March 1866	Arm	Worth 2, Co. List
4	9 Nov 1866 16 April 1867	Leg	Worth 4, Co. List Aud. 6.1, p. 37
5	22 June 1866 (2)	Leg	Jewett Invoices Aud. 6.1, p. 34
6	5 March 1867	Arm	Aud. 6.1, p. 35
7	12 Feb 1866 23 Aug 1866 1 Sept 1866	Leg	Worth 1, letter Worth 3, form Aud. 6.1, p. 34
8	24 Sept 1866 12 Oct 1866	Leg	Worth 3, pwr atty Aud. 6.1, p. 35
9	26 March 1866	Leg	Worth 2, Co. List
10	3 April 1866 26 Feb 1867 27 Feb 1867	Arm	Worth 2, Co. List CW Military 41 Aud. 6.1, p. 35
11	30 Oct 1867 8 Nov 1867	Arm	CW Military 41 Aud. 6.1, p. 33
12	24 Feb 1866	Arm	Worth 1, Co. List
13	9 March 1867 19 March 1867	Leg	Jewett Invoices Aud. 6.1, p. 35
14	no date 16 March 1867	Arm	Worth 8, Co. List Aud. 6.1, p. 36
15	4 May 1867 8 May 1867 11 May 1867 18 May 1867	Arm	CW Military 41 Aud. 6.1, p. 37 CW Military 41 CW Military 41
16	14 Nov 1866 27 Nov 1866 (2)	Leg	CW Military 41 Jewett Invoices Aud. 6.1, p. 35
17	13 March 1866	Arm	Worth 2, Co. List

	Claimant	County	Confederate Unit
1	Munday, J. F. (2) (also Monday)	Catawba	Co. K, 23rd NCT
2	Munn, D. A. (2)	Montgomery	Co. K, 34th NCT
3	Murph, Jacob R. (2) (Joseph in Aud. 6.1)	Stanly	Co. B, 7th NCT
4	Murphy, James M. (3)	Franklin	Co. B, 66th NCT
5	Murphy, John F. (4) (J. L. on Co. List)	Gaston	Co. B, 28th NCT
6	Murry, Thomas O. (2)	Beaufort	Co. C, 4th NCST
7	Myers, J. T. (4) (also Meyers)	Duplin and Sampson	Co. C, 38th NCT
8	Myrick, Benjamin	Halifax	
9	Myrick, M. E.	Moore	Co. E, 26th NCT
10	Nall, Irvin (4) (also Ervin)	Chatham	Co. E, 26th NCT
11	Nance, Richard (2)	Surry	Co. A, 28th NCT
12	Nants, David (3) (also Nantz)	Mecklenburg	Co. C, 37th NCT
13	Nash, Fred[erick, Jr.], Capt. (3)	Orange	[Co. G, 27th NCT]
14	Nash, Thomas J. (2)	Rowan	Co. B, 7th NCST

	Date	Limb	Location
1	24 April 1867 1 Aug 1867	Arm	Aud. 6.1, p. 37 CW Military 41
2	6 Feb 1867 (2)	Leg	Jewett Invoices Aud. 6.1, p. 34
3	5 June 1867 7 June 1867	Arm	CW Military 41 Aud. 6.1, p. 38
4	20 May 1869 22 May 1869 (2)	Arm	CW Military 41 TC $ Bk 4, p. 247 Aud. 6.1, p. 52
5	no date 11 July 1866 20 Nov 1866 (2)	Leg	Worth 8, Co. List Worth 3, letter Jewett Invoices Aud. 6.1, p. 34
6	12 Dec 1866 (2)	Leg	Jewett Invoices Aud. 6.1, p. 34
7	27 Aug 1866 6 Oct 1866 19 Oct 1866 (2)	Leg	Worth 3, form AG 58, p. 155 Jewett Invoices Aud. 6.1, p. 34
8	5 March 1866	Arm	Worth 2, Co. List
9	25 April 1867	Arm	Aud. 6.1, p. 37
10	5 Dec 1866 12 Feb 1867 2 April 1867 (2)	Leg	Worth 4, Co. List CW Military 41 Jewett Invoices Aud. 6.1, p. 39
11	23 Feb 1867 (2)	Arm	CW Military 41 Aud. 6.1, p. 39
12	9 Nov 1866 10 Jan 1868 (2)	Leg	Worth 4, Co. List Worth 8, form Aud. 6.1, p. 39
13	9 Aug 1866 10 Sept 1866 19 Sept 1866	Leg	AG 58, p. 62 Aud. 6.1, p. 39 Jewett Invoices
14	23 April 1866 6 March 1867	Arm	CW Mil, Co. List Aud. 6.1, p. 39

	Claimant	County	Confederate Unit
1	Naylor, Joseph	Sampson	Co. E, 2nd NCST
2	Neal, G. A.	Mecklenburg	Co. E, 11th NCT
3	Neal, J. C. (2)	Cleveland	Co. G, 49th NCT
4	Neel, George	Mecklenburg	[Co. E, 11th NCT]
5	Nelson, George W. (3)	Rockingham	Co. D, 45th NCT
6	Nelson, James R. (3)	Edgecombe and Martin	
7	Nelson, William (3)	Wilkes	Co. K, 53rd NCT
8	Newell, Thomas (3)	Guilford	Co. F, 54th NCT
9	Newsom, H. T. (2)	Stokes	[Co. K, 48th NCT]
10	Newsome, Ensley	Randolph	[Co. I, 2nd NCST]
11	Newsome, Green (2)	Forsyth	Co. B, 1st Bn. NC Sharpshooters
12	Newton, John A. (4)	Cleveland	Co. F, 34th NCT
13	Nichols, Archibald (2)	Orange	Co. C, 6th NCST
14	Nichols, Moses (3) (also Nicholes)	Johnston	Co. E, 27th NCT
15	Nichols, W. R. (2)	Wake	Co. E, 14th NCT
16	Nix, John (3)	Henderson and McDowell	Co. A, 25th NCT

	Date	Limb	Location
1	26 March 1867	Arm	Aud. 6.1, p. 39
2	26 March 1867	Arm	Aud. 6.1, p. 39
3	16 July 1867 15 Aug 1867	Leg	CW Military 41 Aud. 6.1, p. 39
4	9 Nov 1866	Arm	Worth 4, Co. List
5	5 May 1868 (3)	Leg	Worth 8, letter TC $ Bk 4, p. 89 Aud. 6.1, p. 39
6	17 Nov 1866 27 Sept 1867 (2)	Arm	CW Military 41 Aud. 6.1, p. 39 CW Military 41
7	1 Nov 1866 23 Feb 1867 (2)	Arm	Worth 4, Co. List CW Military 41 Aud. 6.1, p. 39
8	no date 23 July 1867 (2)	Arm	Worth 8, Co. List CW Military 41 Aud. 6.1, p. 39
9	28 May 1867 9 June 1867	Hand	CW Military 41 CW Military 41
10	23 April 1867	Arm	Aud. 6.1, p. 39
11	6 Aug 1867 (2)	Leg	Aud. 6.1, p. 39 Worth 6, form
12	11 Dec 1866 21 Dec 1866 (2) 1 July 1868	Leg	CW Military 41 Aud. 6.1, p. 39 CW Military 41 Holden 1, letter
13	21 Sept 1866 (2)	Leg	Jewett Invoices Aud. 6.1, p. 39
14	5 March 1866 13 June 1866 (2)	Leg	Worth 2, Co. List Jewett Invoices Aud. 6.1, p. 39
15	13 July 1867 (2)	Hand	CW Military 41 Aud. 6.1, p. 39
16	16 April 1866 31 May 1866 21 May 1867	Foot	Worth 2, Co. List Worth 2, Co. List Aud. 6.1, p. 39

	Claimant	County	Confederate Unit
1	Norton, J. P. (5) (leg returned in 1869 for $50 commutation)	Iredell	Co. C, 4th NCST
2	Nunn, Andrew J. (3)	Stokes	Co. F, 21st NCT
3	Oakes, James E. (4) (also Oake)	Guilford	Co. B, 45th NCT
4	Oakes, [James] P.	Davie	[Co. A, 21st NCT]
5	O'Brien, Spencer (4)	Granville	Co. E, 23rd NCT
6	O'Bryant, Thomas (2)	Granville	Co. A, 44th NCT
7	Ogburn, C. J. (3)	Forsyth	Co. D, 57th NCT (incorrectly reported as 7th NCST on invoice)
8	Ogburn, Charles (This is probably C. J.)	Forsyth	
9	O'Neal, Charles (2)	Wilson	Co. G, 5th NCST
10	Orr, D. K.	Mecklenburg	[Co. C, 9th NCST (1st NC Cav.)]
11	Orr, Joseph L.	Mecklenburg	Co. I, 37th NCT
12	Outlaw, John E. (4)	Duplin	Co. A, 43rd NCT
13	Overby, W. W.	Wake	Co. E, 14th NCT
14	Overcash, J. H.	Rowan	Co. K, 7th NCST

	Date	Limb	Location
1	3 April 1866 24 Oct 1866 8 Dec 1866 (2) 26 Jan 1869	Leg	Worth 2, Co. List Worth 3, form Jewett Invoices Aud. 6.1, p. 39 Aud. 6.1, p. 39
2	13 June 1867 25 April 1868 27 April 1868	Leg	CW Military 41 Worth 8, letter Aud. 6.1, p. 39
3	20 Oct 1866 (2) no date (2)	Leg	Jewett Invoices Aud. 6.1, p. 40 Worth 8, Co. List and City List
4	13 March 1866	Arm	Worth 2, Co. List
5	12 March 1866 14 June 1866 28 July 1866 (2)	Leg	Worth 2, Co. List Worth 3, form Jewett Invoices Aud. 6.1, p. 40
6	5 June 1867 6 June 1867	Arm	CW Military 41 Aud. 6.1, p. 40
7	23 June 1866 25 July 1866 (2)	Leg	Worth 3, form Jewett Invoices Aud. 6.1, p. 40
8	8 March 1866	Foot	Worth 2, Co. List
9	16 Jan 1867 (2)	Leg	Jewett Invoices Aud. 6.1, p. 40
10	9 Nov 1866	Feet	Worth 4, Co. List
11	25 March 1867	Arm	Aud. 6.1, p. 40
12	19 April 1866 26 Nov 1866 24 Jan 1867 (2)	Leg	CW Mil, Co. List CW Military 41 Jewett Invoices Aud. 6.1, p. 40
13	6 May 1867	Arm	Aud. 6.1, p. 40
14	29 March 1867	Arm	Aud. 6.1, p. 40

	Claimant	County	Confederate Unit
1	Overcash, Otho C.	Caldwell	Co. I, 7th NCST
2	Overman, William A.	Wilson	Co. D, 2nd NCST
3	Owens, A. A.	Rutherford	Co. C, 15th NCT
4	Owens, Henry C. (2)	Rowan	Co. B, 46th NCT
5	Owens, S. T. (2)	Rutherford	Co. I, 56th NCT
6	Pace, Larry (3)	Johnston	Co. C, 1st NCST
7	Padgett, William A. (2)	Stokes	Co. H, 22nd NCT
8	Page, D. F. (2) (erroneously listed as D. L. Page in Aud. 6.1)	Stokes	Co. H, 53rd NCT
9	Page, G. L. (3)	Stokes	
10	Page, William A. (2)	Stokes	[Co. F, 21st NCT]
11	Paget, Green L. (2)	Stokes	Co. F, 21st NCT
12	Paige, C. G., Capt.	Martin	
13	Palmer, G. W. (3)	Davidson	Co. A, 54th NCT
14	Pankey, James	Rowan	Co. H, 43rd NCT
15	Parker, D. (2)	Jackson	[Co. F], 29th NCT
16	Parker, G. W. (2)	Pitt	Co. D, 44th NCT
17	Parker, James (2)	Buncombe	Co. E, 60th NCT

	Date	Limb	Location
1	23 April 1867	Arm	Aud. 6.1, p. 40
2	29 April 1867	Arm	Aud. 6.1, p. 40
3	16 May 1867	Arm	Aud. 6.1, p. 40
4	25 March 1867 27 March 1867	Hand	CW Military 41 Aud. 6.1, p. 40
5	7 May 1867 (2)	Arm	CW Military 41 Aud. 6.1, p. 40
6	2 March 1867 (2) 11 March 1867	Arm	CW Military 41 Aud. 6.1, p. 43 Worth 4, letter
7	21 Feb 1867 (2)	Leg	Jewett Invoices Aud. 6.1, p. 41
8	6 Aug 1867 (2)	Arm	CW Military 41 Aud. 6.1, p. 43
9	28 Nov 1866 14 Jan 1867 12 Feb 1867	Leg	CW Military 41 Worth 4, letter Aud. 6.1, p. 41
10	14 Jan 1867 12 Feb 1867	Leg	Worth 4, letter Aud. 6.1, p. 42
11	2 Feb 1867 25 July 1867	Leg	CW Military 41 CW Military 41
12	13 Sept 1866	Leg	AG 58, p. 121
13	2 June 1866 6 April 1867 (2)	Arm	Worth 3, form Jewett Invoices Aud. 6.1, p. 42
14	18 March 1867	Arm	Aud. 6.1, p. 42
15	26 Feb 1867 27 Feb 1867	Arm	CW Military 41 Aud. 6.1, p. 42
16	25 Sept 1866 (2)	Leg	Jewett Invoices Aud. 6.1, p. 41
17	10 May 1866 13 March 1867	Arm	Worth 2, Co. List Aud. 6.1, p. 42

	Claimant	County	Confederate Unit
1	Parker, James C. (2)	Pasquotank	Co. A, 8th NCST
2	Parker, John M. (2)	Gaston	Co. H, 52nd NCT
3	Parker, Needham	Johnston	Co. C, 1st NCST
4	Parker, William J. (3)	Henderson	Co. D, 25th NCT
5	Parks, John L. (3)	Cabarrus	Co. B, 20th NCT
6	Parsons, Mulky	Wilkes	
7	Parsons, William M.	Wilkes	Co. K, 53rd NCT
8	Partin, G. W. (2)	Harnett and Wake	Co. D, 26th NCT
9	Pasmore, Travis L. (2)	Macon	Co. K, 9th NCST (1st NC Cav.)
10	Pate, George Badger (3)	Greene	Co. A, 3rd NCST
11	Patterson, Ibson F. (2)	Rowan	Co. A, 20th NCT
12	Patterson, J. R. (3)	Buncombe	Co. K, 25th NCT
13	Patterson, John A.	Davie	Co. F, 13th NCT
14	Patterson, John M. (3)	Iredell	Co. A, 29th NCT
15	Patterson, Martin L. (2)	Surry	Co. I, 21st NCT
16	Patterson, Wesley (3)	Transylvania	Co. A, 20th NCT

	Date	Limb	Location
1	7 March 1866 (2)	Leg	Jewett Invoices Aud. 6.1, p. 41
2	4 Sept 1866 (2)	Leg	Aud. 6.1, p. 41 Jewett Invoices
3	2 April 1867	Arm	Aud. 6.1, p. 42
4	2 Aug 1866 24 Oct 1866 (2)	Leg	CW Military 41 Jewett Invoices Aud. 6.1, p. 41
5	26 March 1866 24 Jan 1867 3 Feb 1867	Leg	Worth 2, Co. List CW Military 41 Aud. 6.1, p. 41
6	11 April 1866	Arm	Worth 2, Co. List
7	10 March 1868	Arm	Aud. 6.1, p. 43
8	15 May 1867 no date	Arm	Aud. 6.1, p. 43 CW Mil, Co. List
9	9 July 1867 3 Aug 1867	Arm	CW Military 41 CW Military 41
10	21 Feb 1866 18 March 1867 23 March 1867	Arm	Worth 1, Co. List CW Military 41 Aud. 6.1, p. 42
11	23 April 1866 29 March 1867	Arm	CW Mil, Co. List Aud. 6.1, p. 42
12	10 May 1866 23 March 1867 1 April 1867	Arm	Worth 2, Co. List CW Military 41 Aud. 6.1, p. 42
13	6 May 1868	Hand	CW Military 41
14	3 April 1866 20 Nov 1866 (2)	Leg	Worth 2, Co. List Jewett Invoices Aud. 6.1, p. 41
15	12 Nov 1866 19 Nov 1866	Leg	Worth 4, letter Aud. 6.1, p. 41
16	26 Nov 1867 10 Dec 1867 15 Dec 1867	Leg	Worth 7, form Aud. 6.1, p. 43 CW Military 41

	Claimant	County	Confederate Unit
1	Patterson, Willie T. (2)	Orange	Co. G, 27th NCT
2	Patton, J. M. (4)	Buncombe	Co. E, 60th NCT
3	Paysour, D. R. (3)	Gaston	Co. B, 28th NCT
4	Peace, George T. (4)	Granville	Co. E, 23rd NCT
5	Peaden, John R. (5)	Pitt	Co. F, 61st NCT
6	Pearce, Enoc.	Franklin	Co. C, 66th NCT
7	Peddy, John A.	Wake	Co. I, 41st NCT (3rd NC Cav.)
8	Peel, Turner (2)	Edgecombe	Co. B, 33rd NCT
9	Pence, Noah Franklin (2) (erroneously listed as L. F. Pence in Aud. 6.1)	Stanly	Co. I, 52nd NCT
10	Pendergrass, R. J. (2)	Warren	Co. A, 14th NCT
11	Perkins, Jacob (4)	Richmond	Co. D, 33rd NCT
12	Perry, Henry (3)	Wake	Co. I, 1st NCST
13	Peterson, C. W.	Halifax	Co. A, 14th NCT

	Date	Limb	Location
1	4 May 1867 14 May 1867	Leg	CW Military 41 Aud. 6.1, p. 43
2	10 May 1866 12 Dec 1866 1 Jan 1867 (2)	Leg	Worth 2, Co. List CW Military 41 Jewett Invoices Aud. 6.1, p. 41
3	no date 5 Aug 1867 2 Oct 1867	Arm	Worth 8, Co. List CW Military 41 Aud. 6.1, p. 43
4	12 March 1866 14 June 1866 20 July 1866 (2)	Leg	Worth 2, Co. List Worth 3, form Jewett Invoices Aud. 6.1, p. 41
5	20 Nov 1867 8 Jan 1868 11 Jan 1868 17 Jan 1868 12 Feb 1868	Leg	CW Military 41 Worth 8, letter Worth 8, letter Aud. 6.1, p. 43 CW Military 41
6	20 June 1867	Arm	Aud. 6.1, p. 43
7	7 May 1867	Arm	Aud. 6.1, p. 42
8	12 Dec 1866 (2)	Leg	Jewett Invoices Aud. 6.1, p. 41
9	24 Feb 1866 15 April 1867	Arm	Worth 1, Co. List Aud. 6.1, p. 42
10	28 Aug 1867 (2)	Hand	CW Military 41 Aud. 6.1, p. 43
11	11 April 1866 22 Sept 1866 9 Oct 1866 (2)	Leg	Worth 2, Co. List AG 58, p. 137 Jewett Invoices Aud. 6.1, p. 41
12	18 Jan 1868 (2) no date	Arm	CW Military 41 Aud. 6.1, p. 43 CW Mil, Co. List
13	6 June 1867	Arm	Aud. 6.1, p. 43

	Claimant	County	Confederate Unit
1	Petigrew, Franklin (4) (also Pettigrew)	Rockingham	Co. K, 13th NCT
2	Petteway, John	Onslow	Co. A, 35th NCT
3	Peugh, John H. (3)	New Hanover	Co. F, 3rd NCST
4	Philbeck, J. P. (2)	Cleveland	Co. B, 24th NCT
5	Phillips, Benjamin A.	Yadkin	[Co. F, 28th NCT]
6	Phillips, Wyatt J. (3)	Lenoir	Co. C, 66th NCT
7	Philmon, Elijah K. (5)	Union	Co. A, 27th NCT
8	Pickett, Henry (2)	Orange	Co. G, 27th NCT
9	Pierce, James (2)	Rockingham	Co. K, 45th NCT
10	Pierce, O. H. (2) (also Peirce)	Randolph	Co. H, 38th NCT
11	Pierce, Sampson (4) (also Pearce and Peirce)	Duplin	Co. I, 9th NCST (1st NC Cav.)
12	Piercy, Wesley M. (3) (also Pearcey and Pircee)	Caldwell	Co. I, 26th NCT
13	Pittillo, John L. (3)	Henderson	Co. D, 60th NCT

	Date	Limb	Location
1	12 March 1866 29 June 1867 19 July 1867 6 Aug 1867	Leg	CW Mil, Co. List CW Military 41 Aud. 6.1, p. 43 CW Military 41
2	26 March 1867	Arm	Aud. 6.1, p. 42
3	18 March 1867 19 March 1867 22 March 1867	Arm	CW Military 41 Aud. 6.1, p. 42 CW Military 41
4	23 March 1867 8 April 1867	Leg	CW Military 41 Aud. 6.1, p. 42
5	3 June 1867	Arm	Aud. 6.1, p. 43
6	20 March 1866 25 April 1867 (2)	Arm	Worth 2, Co. List Jewett Invoices Aud. 6.1, p. 42
7	22 Aug 1866 22 Oct 1866 (2) May 1867 21 Dec 1868	Leg	Worth 3, form CW Military 41 Worth 3, Co. List Jewett Invoices Aud. 6.1, p. 41
8	3 Aug 1866 (2)	Leg	Jewett Invoices Aud. 6.1, p. 41
9	3 June 1867 (2)	Leg	CW Military 41 Aud. 6.1, p. 43
10	21 Nov 1866 (2)	Leg	Jewett Invoices Aud. 6.1, p. 41
11	19 April 1866 26 Nov 1866 1 Feb 1867 31 July 1867	Leg	CW Mil, Co. List CW Military 41 Aud. 6.1, p. 41 CW Military 41
12	7 July 1866 8 Jan 1867 (2)	Leg	Worth 3, form Jewett Invoices Aud. 6.1, p. 41
13	16 April 1866 19 Oct 1867 4 Dec 1867	Arm	Worth 2, Co. List Worth 7, form Aud. 6.1, p. 43

	Claimant	County	Confederate Unit
1	Plummer, Jesse B. (6) (leg returned in 1869 for $50 commutation)	Ashe	Co. K, 37th NCT
2	Pollard, Alfred (3)	Wake	[Co. C], 38th Tenn.
3	Ponder, Joseph	Madison	[Co. D, 29th NCT]
4	Pope, Josiah	Sampson	Co. F, 20th NCT
5	Pope, Owen (4)	Union	Co. F, 48th NCT
6	Pope, Reddick (5)	Union	Co. I, 53rd NCT
7	Potts, L[awson] A.	Mecklenburg	[Co. C, 37th NCT]
8	Powell, James J. (2)	Wake	Co. A, 10th NCST (1st NC Arty.)
9	Powell, James W.	Wake	Co. I, 1st NCST
10	Powers, Jordan (3)	Columbus	Co. H, 51st NCT
11	Pratt, George W. (2)	Rockingham	Co. D, 45th NCT
12	Presnel, Wesley	Watauga	Co. I, 58th NCT
13	Presnell, E. L.	Alexander	Co. A, 37th NCT
14	Prestley, Jason (2) (also Preseby)	Buncombe	Co. I, 6th NCST

	Date	Limb	Location
1	7 April 1866 16 June 1866 14 July 1866 16 July 1866 15 Feb 1869 (2)	Leg	Worth 2, Co. List CW Military 41 Jewett Invoices Aud. 6.1, p. 40 TC $ Bk 4, p. 199 Aud. 6.1, p. 43
2	18 June 1866 21 July 1866 (2)	Leg	Worth 3, form Jewett Invoices Aud. 6.1, p. 41
3	28 Feb 1867	Arm	Aud. 6.1, p. 42
4	30 April 1867	Arm	Aud. 6.1, p. 42
5	22 Oct 1866 8 May 1867 11 May 1867 20 May 1867	Arm	Worth 3, Co. List CW Military 41 Aud. 6.1, p. 43 CW Military 41
6	21 July 1866 27 Aug 1866 20 Sept 1866 (2) 22 Oct 1866	Leg	Worth 3, form AG 58, p. 91 Jewett Invoices Aud. 6.1, p. 41 Worth 3, Co. List
7	9 Nov 1866	Arm	Worth 4, Co. List
8	30 May 1867 31 May 1867	Leg	Aud. 6.1, p. 43 CW Military 41
9	19 Aug 1867	Arm	Aud. 6.1, p. 43
10	12 May 1867 1 June 1867 no date	Arm	CW Military 41 Aud. 6.1, p. 43 CW Military 41
11	12 March 1866 5 April 1867	Arm	CW Mil, Co. List Aud. 6.1, p. 42
12	28 Feb 1867	Arm	Aud. 6.1, p. 42
13	29 Nov 1867	Arm	Aud. 6.1, p. 43
14	10 May 1866 15 April 1867	Leg	Worth 2, Co. List Aud. 6.1, p. 42

	Claimant	County	Confederate Unit
1	Price, E. G., Capt. (3)	Martin	Co. B, 33rd NCT
2	Price, James T.	Anson	Co. I, 43rd NCT
3	Price, James T. (3)	Johnston	Co. C, 5th NCST
4	Price, John M. M. (2)	Rutherford	Co. I, 56th NCT
5	Price, Thomas	Anson	[Co. I, 43rd NCT]
6	Price, W. H.	Anson	Co. I, 43rd NCT
7	Pridgeon, Drewry	Nash	Co. I, 30th NCT
8	Propst, John (2)	Catawba	Co. G, 57th NCT
9	Puckett, Hugh (2)	Surry	[Co. A, 28th NCT]
10	Puryear, D. H.	Granville	
11	Puryear, Henry Y. (2)	Granville	Co. I, 23rd NCT
12	Putnam, Samuel (3) (also Putman and Pulman)	Cleveland	Co. D, 49th NCT (2nd Co. B. in *NCT Roster*)
13	Putnam, William A. (4) (also Pulman)	Cleveland	Co. B, 49th NCT
14	Quate, Richard (4) (also Quait)	Guilford	Co. C, 45th NCT
15	Queen, R. B. (2)	Wilkes	Co. G, 37th NCT
16	Quinn, David (4)	Lenoir	Co. D, 27th NCT

	Date	Limb	Location
1	4 July 1866 20 Sept 1866 (2)	Leg	Worth 3, form Jewett Invoices Aud. 6.1, p. 41
2	7 May 1867	Leg	Aud. 6.1, p. 42
3	5 March 1866 15 June 1866 (2)	Leg	Worth 2, Co. List Jewett Invoices Aud. 6.1, p. 41
4	5 June 1867 (2)	Leg	CW Military 41 Aud. 6.1, p. 43
5	1 May 1867	Leg	CW Military 41
6	7 May 1867	Arm	Aud. 6.1, p. 42
7	13 April 1867	Arm	Aud. 6.1, p. 42
8	22 April 1867 25 April 1867	Arm	CW Military Aud. 6.1, p. 42
9	26 May 1866 1 June 1866	Leg	Worth 2, letter Aud. 6.1, p. 41
10	12 March 1866	Arm	Worth 2, Co. List
11	16 May 1867 28 May 1867	Arm	CW Military 41 Aud. 6.1, p. 43
12	no date 12 March 1867 13 March 1867	Arm	Worth 8, Co. List CW Military 41 Aud. 6.1, p. 42
13	no date 23 Nov 1866 20 Dec 1866 (2)	Leg	Worth 8, Co. List CW Military 41 Jewett Invoices Aud. 6.1, p. 41
14	no date (2) 13 Oct 1866 (2)	Leg	Worth 8, Co. List and City List Jewett Invoices Aud. 6.1, p. 44
15	21 June 1867	Hand	CW Military 41
16	20 March 1866 24 Aug. 1866 17 Sept 1866 (2)	Leg	Worth 2, Co. List AG 58, p. 86 Jewett Invoices Aud. 6.1, p. 44

	Claimant	County	Confederate Unit
1	Quinn, Henry O. (4)	New Hanover	Co. C, 1st NC
2	Rabb, George W. (6)	Catawba	Co. A, 12th NCT
3	Rabb, William M. (2)	Cleveland	Co. K. 49th NCT
4	Rabon, Jonathan	Davie	Co. E, 42nd NCT
5	Rains, William C. (2)	Polk	Co. I, 54th NCT
6	Ramsay, William S.	Chatham	Co. D, 61st NCT
7	Ramsour, T. J. (2)	Lincoln	Co. I, 11th NCT
8	Randall—see also Randolph		
9	Randall, J. C. (2)	Cleveland	[Co. D, 14th NCT]
10	Randolph, Elijah (3) (also Elish Randolph and Elijah Randall)	Yancey	[Co. C, 16th NCT]
11	Ranies, William C.	Polk	Co. I, 54th NCT
12	Rankin, William H. (3)	Guilford	Co. I, 21st NCT
13	Rape, Henry N. (3)	Union	Co. D, 37th NCT
14	Ray, Abner	Rowan	Co. H, 24th NCT

	Date	Limb	Location
1	4 April 1867 22 April 1867 25 April 1867 6 May 1867	Leg	CW Military 41 Worth 5, form Aud. 6.1, p. 44 CW Military 41
2	24 Feb 1866 24 May 1866 8 Jan 1867 (2) 15 Feb 1867 25 Feb 1868	Leg	Worth 1, Co. List Worth 2, form Jewett Invoices Aud. 6.1, p. 45 CW Military 41 CW Military 41
3	10 Oct 1867 (2)	Hand	CW Military 41 Aud. 6.1, p. 47
4	18 July 1867	Arm	Aud. 6.1, p. 47
5	17 April 1866 22 July 1867	Arm	Worth 2, Co. List Aud. 6.1, p. 47
6	21 Feb 1867	Arm	Aud. 6.1, p. 45
7	13 June 1866 (2)	Leg	Jewett Invoices Aud. 6.1, p. 45
8			
9	14 March 1867 19 March 1867	Arm	CW Military 41 Aud. 6.1, p. 46
10	7 April 1866 31 Aug 1867 2 Oct 1867	Arm	Worth 2, Co. List CW Military 41 Aud. 6.1, p. 47
11	15 July 1867	Arm	CW Military 41
12	no date 3 Nov 1866 (2)	Leg	Worth 8, City List Jewett Invoices Aud. 6.1, p. 45
13	1 July 1867 6 July 1867 22 July 1867	Hand	Worth 6, letter Aud. 6.1, p. 47 CW Military 41
14	5 March 1868	Arm	Aud. 6.1, p. 47

	Claimant	County	Confederate Unit
1	Ray, N. W. (4)	Cumberland	[Co. D, 6th NCST]
2	Raybond, Jonathan	Davie	
3	Rea, James	Mecklenburg	[Co. H, 35th NCT]
4	Redmond, James	Orange	Co. C, 6th NCST
5	Redmond, Thaddeus	Orange	Co. C, 5th NCST (6th NCST in NCT *Roster*)
6	Reed, A. J. (7) (also Reid)	Alexander	Co. G, 37th NCT
7	Reid, W. J.	Alexander	Co. B, 19th NCT (2nd NC Cav.)
8	Reid, William F. (4)	Guilford	Co. B, 21st NCT
9	Reitzel, Henry J. (5)	Catawba	Co. A, 12th NCT
10	Reynolds, John H. (3) (also Reynols)	Haywood and Buncombe	[Co. F, 60th NCT]
11	Reynolds, Lawson	Gaston	Co. H, 23rd NCT
12	Rhea, James (3)	Mecklenburg	Co. H, 37th NCT

	Date	Limb	Location
1	29 May 1866 25 June 1866 27 June 1866 27 July 1866	Leg	CW Military 41 Aud. 6.1, p. 45 AG 58, p. 35 CW Military 41
2	9 May 1867	Arm	CW Military 41
3	9 Nov 1866	Wrist	Worth 4, Co. List
4	19 April 1867	Leg	Aud. 6.1, p. 46
5	23 April 1867	Arm	Aud. 6.1, p. 46
6	2 July 1866 5 July 1866 16 July 1866 20 July 1866 27 Aug 1866 30 Aug 1866 (2)	Leg	CW Military 41 AG 58, p. 38 AG 58, p. 48 AG 58, p. 103 Aud. 6.1, p. 45 Jewett Invoices
7	18 April 1867	Arm	Aud. 6.1, p. 46
8	18 Oct 1866 (2) no date (2)	Leg	Aud. 6.1, p. 45 Jewett Invoices Worth 8, Co. List and City List
9	24 Feb 1866 30 May 1866 18 June 1866 31 July 1866 (2)	Leg	Worth 1, Co. List Worth 2, letter Worth 3, form Jewett Invoices Aud. 6.1, p. 45
10	15 May 1866 11 June 1867 18 June 1867	Arm	Worth 2, Co. List CW Military 41 Aud. 6.1, p. 46
11	28 Nov 1867	Hip and Knee	CW Military 41
12	17 April 1867 25 April 1867 30 April 1867	Arm	CW Military 41 Aud. 6.1, p. 46 CW Military 41

	Claimant	County	Confederate Unit
1	Rhew, William L.	Wake	Co. K, 19th NCT (2nd NC Cav.)
2	Rhodes, George	Buncombe	[Co. I, 25th NCT]
3	Rhom, Robert H. (3)	McDowell	Co. A, 49th NCT
4	Rhyne, George C. (2)	Gaston	Co. B, 28th NCT
5	Rich, Eleazar	Sampson	Co. G, 55th NCT
6	Richardson, David (5) (leg returned in 1869 for $50 commutation)	Alleghany	Co. I, 61st NCT
7	Richardson, Joshua (4) (spelled Richesson in Worth 2)	Alleghany and Ashe	Co. A, 34th NCT
8	Richardson, S. D. (4)	Union	Co. B, 26th NCT
9	Richardson, William W. (3)	Johnston	Co. C, 24th NCT
10	Riddle, Joseph	Cleveland	Co. G, 49th NCT
11	Riddle, Samuel (4)	Yancey	Co. C, 58th NCT
12	Ridenour, Joseph (2)	Surry	[Co. H], 54th NCT
13	Riggs, Columbus (2)	Surry	Co. A, 28th NCT
14	Riggs, Haywood	Craven	Co. F, 2nd NCST

	Date	Limb	Location
1	19 April 1867	Arm	Aud. 6.1, p. 46
2	10 May 1866	Arm	Worth 2, Co. List
3	31 May 1866	Leg	Worth 2, Co. List
	6 Dec 1866 (2)		Jewett Invoices
			Aud. 6.1, p. 45
4	no date	Arm	Worth 8, Co. List
	27 Feb 1867		Aud. 6.1, p. 46
5	27 March 1867	Arm	Aud. 6.1, p. 47
6	11 Feb 1866 (2)	Leg	Jewett Invoices
			Aud. 6.1, p. 45
	18 Oct 1866		AG 58, p. 183
	24 June 1869 (2)		TC $ Bk 4, p. 257
			Aud. 6.1, p. 45
7	7 April 1866	Arm	Worth 2, Co. List
	23 July 1867		Aud. 6.1, p. 47
	16 Aug 1867		CW Military 41
	29 Aug 1867		CW Military 41
8	22 Oct 1866	Arm	Worth 3, Co. List
	14 March 1867		CW Military 41
	27 March 1867		Aud. 6.1, p. 46
	12 April 1867		CW Military 41
9	2 April 1868	Leg	Worth 8, letter
	4 April 1868		Worth 8, letter
	6 April 1868		Aud. 6.1, p. 47
10	8 April 1867	Arm	Aud. 6.1, p. 46
11	7 April 1866	Leg	Worth 2, Co. List
	1 Dec 1866		CW Military 41
	8 Feb 1867 (2)		Jewett Invoices
			Aud. 6.1, p. 45
12	23 Feb 1867 (2)	Arm	CW Military 41
			Aud. 6.1, p. 45
13	23 Feb 1867 (2)	Arm	CW Military 41
			Aud. 6.1, p. 47
14	13 May 1867	Arm	Aud. 6.1, p. 46

	Claimant	County	Confederate Unit
1	Riley, James (4)	Orange	Co. D, 56th NCT
2	Riley, Nathaniel (5)	Person	Co. K, 55th NCT
3	Riley, Vinson	Guilford	Co. E, 22nd NCT
4	Rivenbark, Robert (3)	New Hanover	Co. K, 3rd NCST
5	Roach, James T. (3)	Rockingham	Co. G, 45th NCT
6	Roberson, Jesse	Martin	Co. F, 31st NCT
7	Roberts, ⸺	Wake	
8	Roberts, Anderson (3) (also Robberts)	Alamance	Co. K, 6th NCST
9	Roberts, Charles M. (2)	Granville	Cos. [E and] B, [9th NCST (1st NC Cav.)]
10	Roberts, James A.	Gates	Co. H, 68th NCT
11	Roberts, James [P.]	Cleveland	[Co. I, 68th NCT]
12	Roberts, William H.	Wake	Co. G, 23rd NCT
13	Roberts, Zachariah (2)	Wake	Co. I, 6th NCST
14	Robertson, J. F. M.	Rockingham	Co. H, 13th NCT
15	Robeson, Archibald (6) (also Robertson)	Columbus	Co. C, 20th NCT

	Date	Limb	Location
1	28 June 1866 17 Nov 1866 (2) no date	Leg	CW Military 41 Jewett Invoices Aud. 6.1, p. 45 CW Military 41
2	27 Sept 1866 18 Oct 1866 6 Nov 1866 (2) 27 Nov 1866	Leg	Worth 3, form AG 58, p. 182 Jewett Invoices Aud. 6.1, p. 45 Worth 4, Co. List
3	no date	Arm	Worth 8, Co. List
4	4 April 1867 9 April 1867 15 April 1867	Arm	CW Military 41 Aud. 6.1, p. 46 CW Military 41
5	12 March 1866 10 Aug 1866 13 Aug 1866	Leg	CW Mil, Co. List Worth 3, form Aud. 6.1, p. 45
6	21 Feb 1867	Arm	Aud. 6.1, p. 45
7	no date	Arm	CW Mil, Co. List
8	24 April 1867 26 April 1867 3 May 1867	Arm	CW Military 41 Aud. 6.1, p. 46 CW Military 41
9	12 March 1866 19 June 1867	Leg	Worth 2, Co. List Aud. 6.1, p. 46
10	15 April 1868	Arm	Aud. 6.1, p. 47
11	24 Aug 1867	Finger	CW Military 41
12	21 Feb 1867	Arm	Aud. 6.1, p. 45
13	20 Nov 1867 21 Nov 1867	Hand	CW Military 41 Aud. 6.1, p. 47
14	7 Nov 1866	Leg	Aud. 6.1, p. 45
15	12 Jan 1867 8 March [1867] 16 March 1867 17 March 1867 23 March 1867 May 1867	Leg	Jewett Invoices CW Military 41 Aud. 6.1, p. 45 CW Military 41 CW Military 41 Jewett Invoices

	Claimant	County	Confederate Unit
1	Robeson, S. B.	Mecklenburg	
2	Robeson, W. W.	Mecklenburg	
3	Robinson, Josiah (2)	Sampson	Co. C, 51st NCT
4	Rochell, A. Hiram (2) (also High)	Wake	Co. I, 47th NCT
5	Rodgers, Francis L. (3) (also Rogers)	Union	Co. B, 15th NCT
6	Rodgers, Martin	Rowan	
7	Rogers, Wesley	Wake	
8	Rogers, Western R. (2) (also Rodgers)	Wake	Co. C, 47th NCT
9	Rogers, Wilson	Mecklenburg	
10	Ross, John (3)	Union	Co. F, 35th NCT
11	Ross, T. M.	Pitt	Co. E, 66th NCT
12	Rouse, Thomas J. (3)	Craven	Co. F, 2nd NCST
13	Rowe, Thomas J. (2)	Wilson	Co. A, 16th Bn. NC Cav.
14	Rowe, William (5)	Wilson	Co. C, 43rd NCT
15	Rowland, J. M.	Wake	Co. I, 5th NCST
16	Rowland, James H. (3)	Granville	Co. E, 23rd NCT
17	Royal, H. S. (2)	Sampson	Co. A, 30th NCT

	Date	Limb	Location
1	9 Nov 1866	Leg	Worth 4, Co. List
2	9 Nov 1866	Foot	Worth 4, Co. List
3	2 July 1867 3 July 1867	Leg	CW Military 41 Aud. 6.1, p. 47
4	no date 8 March 1867	Arm	CW Mil, Co. List Aud. 6.1, p. 46
5	22 Oct 1866 25 Feb 1867 (2)	Arm	Worth 3, Co. List CW Military 41 Aud. 6.1, p. 46
6	23 April 1866	Leg	CW Mil, Co. List
7	no date	Arm	CW Mil, Co. List
8	1 March 1867 (2)	Arm	CW Military 41 Aud. 6.1, p. 46
9	9 Nov 1866	Leg	Worth 4, Co. List
10	22 Oct 1866 25 Feb 1867 (2)	Arm	Worth 3, Co. List CW Military 41 Aud. 6.1, p. 45
11	8 March 1867	Arm	Aud. 6.1, p. 46
12	16 Aug 1866 19 Oct 1866 (2)	Leg	Worth 3, form Jewett Invoices Aud. 6.1, p. 45
13	16 Jan 1867 (2)	Leg	Jewett Invoices Aud. 6.1, p. 45
14	9 April 1867 25 April 1867 7 May 1867 23 May 1867 11 June 1867	Arm	CW Military 41 Aud. 6.1, p. 46 CW Military 41 CW Military 41 CW Military 41
15	19 May 1867	Arm	Aud. 6.1, p. 46
16	12 March 1866 13 May 1867 28 May 1867	Arm	Worth 2, Co. List CW Military 41 Aud. 6.1, p. 46
17	16 Oct 1866 (2)	Leg	Jewett Invoices Aud. 6.1, p. 45

	Claimant	County	Confederate Unit
1	Royal, S., Lt.	Sampson	
2	Royster, D. W. (2)	Wake	Co. K, 14th NCT
3	Royster, George W. (3)	Granville	Co. D, 12th NCT
4	Rudisill, Henry P. (2)	Catawba	Co. A, 12th NCT
5	Runnels, Laswon	Gaston	Co. H, 23rd NCT
6	Russ, John J. (5)	Robeson	Co. D, 18th NCT
7	Russell, W. H.	Granville	Co. E, 23rd NCT
8	Ruth, Robert	Wake	
9	Ruth, Rufus H. (2)	Wake	Co. K, 14th NCT
10	Safley, William W. (2) (also Safely)	Stanly	Co. D, 28th NCT
11	Sain, Andrew (3)	Lincoln	Co. G, 57th NCT
12	Salmon, Joseph (2)	Cumberland and New Hanover	Co. B, 56th NCT
13	Salmons, William (2)	Bladen	Co. H, 3rd NCST
14	Sanford, Samuel	Rowan	Co. F, 7th NCST
15	Sarratt, U. (2)	Cleveland	Co. C, 15th NCT
16	Sasser, Ira S.	Columbus	Co. H, 18th NCT

	Date	Limb	Location
1	5 Oct 1866		AG 58, p. 151
2	6 June 1867 (2)	Arm	CW Military 41 Aud. 6.1, p. 46
3	12 March 1866 20 June 1867 3 July 1867	Arm	Worth 2, Co. List CW Military 41 Aud. 6.1, p. 47
4	24 Feb 1866 23 April 1867	Arm	Worth 1, Co. List Aud. 6.1, p. 46
5	31 Dec 1867		CW Military 41
6	21 Feb 1866 4 July 1866 10 Oct 1866 21 Nov 1866 (2)	Leg	Worth 1, Co. List Worth 3, form Worth 3, Co. List Jewett Invoices Aud. 6.1, p. 45
7	6 Sept 1867	Arm	Aud. 6.1, p. 47
8	no date	Shoulder	CW Mil, Co. List
9	21 Feb 1867 (2)	Arm	CW Military 41 Aud. 6.1, p. 45
10	24 Feb 1866 14 Dec 1866 (2)	Leg	Worth 1, Co. List Jewett Invoices Aud. 6.1, p. 48
11	12 Oct 1866 24 Oct 1866 (2)	Leg	AG 58, p. 169 Jewett Invoices Aud. 6.1, p. 48
12	22 May 1867 2 Feb 1868	Arm	Aud. 6.1, p. 51 CW Military 41
13	4 June 1867 5 June 1867	Leg	CW Military 41 Aud. 6.1, p. 41
14	24 June 1867	Arm	CW Military 41
15	12 March 1867 16 March 1867	Arm	CW Military 41 Aud. 6.1, p. 50
16	13 Jan 1867	Foot	Aud. 6.1, p. 49

	Claimant	County	Confederate Unit
1	Sawyer, Samuel L. (6)	Tyrrell	Co. A, 32nd NCT
2	Scoggin, Nathan	Cleveland	
3	Scott, Blaney (2)	Wayne	Co. A, 55th NCT
4	Scott, Franklin	Davidson	Co. A, 21st NCT
5	Scott, George W.	Orange	Co. E, 31st NCT
6	Scott, James C.	Orange	Co. B, 6th NCST
7	Scott, William D. (4)	Person	Co. D, 13th NCT
8	Scroggs, Amos (3) (also Scruggs)	Iredell	Co. C, 48th NCT (erroneously reported as Co. E in Aud.)
9	Scroggs, William A. (2)	Macon	Co. I, 39th NCT
10	Seagle, P. C. (4)	Lincoln	Co. B, 23rd NCT
11	Sechler, James P. (2)	Rowan	Co. G, 42nd NCT
12	Segraves, C.	Wake	Co. G, 1st NCST
13	Shankle, C. A. (2)	Stanly	Co. H, 14th NCT
14	Sharp, George V. (2) (also Sharpe)	Rockingham	Co. F, 45th NCT
15	Shaw, Daniel (2)	Columbus	Co. G, 51st NCT

	Date	Limb	Location
1	26 Feb 1866 20 Feb 1867 7 Dec 1867 11 Dec 1867 (2) 24 Dec 1867	Arm	Worth 1, letter CW Military 41 CW Military 41 CW Military 41 Aud. 6.1, p. 52 CW Military 41
2	8 May 1867		CW Military 41
3	10 May 1867 11 May 1867	Arm	CW Military 41 Aud. 6.1, p. 51
4	4 May 1867	Arm	Aud. 6.1, p. 52
5	9 April 1867	Arm	Aud. 6.1, p. 50
6	11 April 1867	Arm	Aud. 6.1, p. 50
7	29 May 1866 9 Nov 1866 (2) 27 Nov 1866	Leg	Worth 2, form Jewett Invoices Aud. 6.1, p. 49 Worth 4, Co. List
8	3 April 1866 20 Nov 1866 (2)	Leg	Worth 2, Co. List Jewett Invoices Aud. 6.1, p. 49
9	28 Jan 1867 (2)	Leg	CW Military 41 Aud. 6.1, p. 49
10	15 Sept 1866 12 Oct 1866 7 Nov 1866 (2)	Leg	Worth 3, letter AG 58, p. 166 Jewett Invoices Aud. 6.1, p. 48
11	23 April 1866 26 April 1867	Arm	CW Mil, Co. List Aud. 6.1, p. 51
12	19 May 1867	Arm	Aud. 6.1, p. 51
13	2 Aug 1867 (2)	Arm	CW Military 41 Aud. 6.1, p. 52
14	8 July 1867 6 Aug 1867	Ankle	CW Military 41 Aud. 6.1, p. 52
15	26 Feb 1867 (2)	Arm	CW Military 41 Aud. 6.1, p. 49

	Claimant	County	Confederate Unit
1	Shaw, W. H. H. (2)	Wake	Co. E, 14th NCT
2	Shearin, M. L. (4) (also Shearrin)	Halifax	Co. I, 12th NCT
3	Sherran, William (2) (also Sherrand) (loss of arm erroneously reported in Aud.)	Wake	Co. A, 44th NCT
4	Sherrill, J. A.	Lincoln	Co. G, 52nd NCT
5	Sherrill, M. L.	Halifax	Co. I, 12th NCT
6	Sherrill, Miles O. (3)	Catawba	Co. A, 12th NCT
7	Shipp, N. M. (2)	Wake	Co. I, 6th NCST
8	Shoe, Henry (2)	Guilford	Co. E, 28th NCT
9	Shook, Jacob A. (2)	Burke	Co. B, 54th NCT
10	Shore, E. H. (3)	Forsyth	Co. I, 33rd NCT
11	Shouse, Wiley (4)	Forsyth	Co. B, 1st Bn. NC Sharpshooters
12	Shull, W. F.	Watauga	Co. E, 37th NCT
13	Shuller, John	Randolph	Co. H, 38th NCT
14	Shultz, C. A. (3)	Forsyth	Co. B, 1st Bn. NC Sharpshooters

	Date	Limb	Location
1	1 June 1867 (2)	Ankle	CW Military 41 Aud. 6.1, p. 51
2	5 March 1866 24 June 1866 22 Sept 1866 26 Sept 1866	Leg	Worth 2, Co. List Worth 3, form AG 58, p. 132 Jewett Invoices
3	4 June 1867 (2)	Leg	CW Military 41 Aud. 6.1, p. 51
4	24 April 1867	Arm	Aud. 6.1, p. 50
5	26 Sept 1866	Leg	Aud. 6.1, p. 48
6	24 Feb 1866 14 Nov 1866 (2)	Leg	Worth 1, Co. List Jewett Invoices Aud. 6.1, p. 48
7	18 April 1867 (2)	Leg	CW Military 41 Aud. 6.1, p. 52
8	no date 16 April 1867	Arm	Worth 8, City List Aud. 6.1, p. 50
9	31 May 1866 1 May 1867	Arm	Worth 2, Co. List Aud. 6.1, p. 51
10	11 April 1867 26 April 1867 8 May 1867	Arm	CW Military 41 Aud. 6.1, p. 51 CW Military 41
11	8 March 1866 25 June 1866 24 July 1866 (2)	Foot	Worth 2, Co. List Worth 3, form Jewett Invoices Aud. 6.1, p. 48
12	28 Feb 1867	Arm	Aud. 6.1, p. 50
13	13 Dec 1867	Arm	Aud. 6.1, p. 52
14	8 March 1866 19 April 1867 26 April 1867	Arm	Worth 2, Co. List CW Military 41 Aud. 6.1, p. 51

	Claimant	County	Confederate Unit
1	Sides, Daniel Simeon (5) (listed as S. D. on invoice)	Cabarrus and Rowan	Co. C, 33rd NCT
2	Sides, H. W. (2)	Stanly	Co. A, 4th NCST
3	Sikes, Henry E. (2)	Cumberland	[Co. A, 5th NCST]
4	Simmons, Alexander (2)	Bladen	Co. A, 18th NCT
5	Simmons, J. S. (4)	Rutherford	Co. H, 9th Ark.
6	Simmons, Pleasant	Rockingham	
7	Simpson, George W. (2)	Alamance	Co. K, 6th NCST
8	Simpson, J. R.	Craven	Co. K, 2nd NCST
9	Simpson, Jacob (2)	Cabarrus	Co. G, 5th NCST
10	Sims, W. M.		Co. D, 56th NCT
11	Sinclair, Albert D. (2)	Anson	[Co. I, 43rd NCT]
12	Sinclair. D. F.	Moore	Co. D, 48th NCT
13	Sinclair, L. A.	Anson	Co. A, 4th NCST
14	Sink, Andrew (2)	Davidson	Co. B, 14th NCT
15	Skidmore, James T. (2)	Gaston	Co. M, 16th NCT
16	Slatton, Jeptha (2)	Jackson	Co. B, 25th NCT
17	Sloan, A. H.	Chatham	Co. B, 61st NCT

	Date	Limb	Location
1	26 March 1866 23 April 1866 6 Nov 1866 (2) 29 March 1867	Leg and Arm	Worth 2, Co. List CW Mil, Co. List Jewett Invoices Aud. 6.1, p. 49 Aud. 6.1, p. 50
2	15 May 1867 (2)	Wrist	CW Military 41 Aud. 6.1, p. 51
3	20 March 1867 21 March 1867	Arm	CW Military 41 Aud. 6.1, p. 50
4	29 May 1867 30 May 1867	Arm	CW Military 41 Aud. 6.1, p. 51
5	10 Sept 1866 12 Oct 1866 23 Oct 1866 (2)	Leg	Worth 3, form AG 58, p. 165 Jewett Invoices Aud. 6.1, p. 48
6	12 March 1866	Arm	CW Mil, Co. List
7	10 March 1866 12 March 1867	Arm	Worth 2, Co. List Aud. 6.1, p. 50
8	24 April 1867	Arm	Aud. 6.1, p. 50
9	26 March 1866 27 March 1867	Arm	Worth 2, Co. List Aud. 6.1, p. 49
10	27 May 1867	Leg	CW Military 41
11	23 March 1867 27 March 1867	Arm	CW Military 41 Aud. 6.1, p. 49
12	23 March 1867	Arm	Aud. 6.1, p. 50
13	1 May 1867	Arm	Aud. 6.1, p. 51
14	8 June 1867 10 June 1867	Arm	CW Military 41 Aud. 6.1, p. 52
15	23 July 1867 (2)	Arm	CW Military 41 Aud. 6.1, p. 52
16	26 Feb 1867 (2)	Arm	CW Military 41 Aud. 6.1, p. 50
17	27 May 1867	Arm	Aud. 6.1, p. 51

	Claimant	County	Confederate Unit
1	Sloan, Frank	Mecklenburg	
2	Sloan, William L. (3)	Mecklenburg	Co. F, 5th NCST
3	Sluder, James (4)	Buncombe	Co. A, 60th NCT
4	Small, Charles W. (3)	Perquimans	Co. C, 2nd NCST
5	Smith, B[enjamin] F.	Stanly	[Co. K, 28th NCT]
6	Smith, C. S. (2)	Rockingham	Co. G, 45th NCT
7	Smith, David	Catawba	[Co. G, 53rd NCT]
8	Smith, E. J. (2)	Stanly	Co. C, 14th NCT
9	Smith, Fred (2)	Chatham	Co. G, 48th NCT
10	Smith, James H. (2)	Wayne	Co. A, 27th NCT
11	Smith, John (2)	Burke	Co. K, 42nd NCT
12	Smith, John J. (4)	Lincoln	Co. I, 11th NCT
13	Smith, John L. (2)	Alleghany	Co. A, 9th NCST (1st NC Cav.)
14	Smith, John W. (3)	Rowan	Co. G, 42nd NCT
15	Smith, P. H. (2)	New Hanover	Co. F, 3rd NCST

	Date	Limb	Location
1	9 Nov 1866	Leg	Worth 4, Co. List
2	23 March 1867 26 March 1867 5 April 1867	Arm	CW Military 41 Aud. 6.1, p. 50 CW Military 41
3	10 May 1866 12 Dec 1866 28 Dec 1866 (2)	Leg	Worth 2, Co. List CW Military 41 Jewett Invoices Aud. 6.1, p. 49
4	March 1866 27 March 1867 24 April 1867	Arm	Worth 2, Co. List CW Military 41 Aud. 6.1, p. 51
5	12 Aug 1867		Worth 6, letter
6	3 June 1867 (2)	Hand	CW Military 41 Aud. 6.1, p. 51
7	24 Feb 1866	Leg	Worth 1, Co. List
8	15 Nov 1866 (2)	Knee	Jewett Invoices Aud. 6.1, p. 48
9	15 June 1867 19 July 1867	Fingers	CW Military 41 Aud. 6.1, p. 52
10	16 Feb 1867 (2)	Leg	Jewett Invoices Aud. 6.1, p. 49
11	9 Jan 1868 (2)	Arm	CW Military 41 Aud. 6.1, p. 52
12	13 Oct 1866 10 Nov 1866 (2) 8 Aug 1867	Leg	AG 58, p. 171 Jewett Invoices Aud. 6.1, p. 48 CW Military 41
13	26 Feb 1867 27 Feb 1867	Arm	CW Military 41 Aud. 6.1, p. 50
14	23 April 1866 4 July 1866 (2)	Leg	CW Mil, Co. List Jewett Invoices Aud. 6.1, p. 48
15	10 Dec 1866 (2) (1867 in Aud. is an error.)	Leg	Jewett Invoices Aud. 6.1, p. 48

	Claimant	County	Confederate Unit
1	Smith, Pinkney R. (3)	Guilford	Co. B, 45th NCT
2	Smith, S. A.	Gaston	Co. H, 5th SC
3	Smith, W. F. (3)	Davie	
4	Smith, William M. (2)	Randolph and Guilford	Co. I, 22nd NCT
5	Smith, William T.	Caswell	
6	Smith, William W. (3)	Union	Co. E, 48th NCT
7	Snider, Thomas L. (4)	Haywood	Co. C, 25th NCT
8	Snipes, William	Wake	Co. D, 26th NCT
9	Snow, John A. (4)	Halifax	Co. G, 12th NC
10	Snuggs, Isaiah (2)	Stanly	Co. H, 14th NCT
11	Soloman, Anderson (2)	Stokes	
12	Somerlin, Owen	Edgecombe	Co. I, 15th NCT
13	Sowell, Eli P. (4)	Moore	Co. H, 26th NCT
14	Spangler, John (2)	Cleveland	Co. F, 55th NCT
15	Sparkman, Jacob	Robeson	

	Date	Limb	Location
1	27 March 1867 no date (2)	Arm	Aud. 6.1, p. 49 Worth 8, Co. List and City List
2	8 April 1867	Leg	Aud. 6.1, p. 50
3	13 March 1866 13 April 1867 (2)	Arm	Worth 2, Co. List Jewett Invoices Aud. 6.1, p. 50
4	29 Oct 1866 7 March 1867	Arm	Worth 3, Co. List Aud. 6.1, p. 50
5	20 Feb 1866	Leg	Worth 1, Co. List
6	22 Oct 1866 29 May 1867 13 June 1867	Arm	Worth 3, Co. List CW Military 41 CW Military 41
7	15 May 1866 15 April 1867 21 June 1867 8 July 1867	Foot	Worth 2, Co. List CW Military 41 Aud. 6.1, p. 52 CW Military 41
8	19 May 1867	Arm	Aud. 6.1, p. 51
9	5 March 1866 5 May 1866 13 April 1868 16 April 1868	Arm	Worth 2, Co. List Worth 2, letter CW Military 41 Aud. 6.1, p. 52
10	23 Nov 1866 (2)	Leg	Jewett Invoices Aud. 6.1, p. 48
11	21 March 1867 20 May 1867	Leg	CW Military 41 Aud. 6.1, p. 51
12	26 Nov 1867	Arm	Aud. 6.1, p. 52
13	16 Feb 1866 27 Feb 1866 (2) 11 July 1866	Leg	Worth 1, form Jewett Invoices Aud. 6.1, p. 48 Worth 3, letter
14	no date 16 March 1867	Arm	Worth 8, Co. List Aud. 6.1, p. 50
15	10 Oct 1866	Leg	Worth 3, Co. List

	Claimant	County	Confederate Unit
1	Spaugh, J. R. (3) (also Spach)	Forsyth	Co. K, 21st NCT
2	Speck, J. F., Capt. (3) (erroneously listed as G. F. in Aud.)	Lincoln	Co. G, 57th NCT
3	Spence, Nathan	Cumberland	Co. E, 44th NCT
4	Spivey, Albert A. (5)	Northampton	Co. D, 54th NCT
5	Spivey, Lewis J. (4)	Robeson	Co. F, 51st NCT
6	Spock, James	Forsyth	
7	Spratt, A. A. (2)	Rutherford	Co. G, 16th NCT
8	Spurling, J. J. (3) (also Spurlin)	Cleveland	Co. F, 56th NCT
9	Stacey, T. F.	Lincoln	Co. G, 16th NCT
10	Stafford, George W. (2)	Davidson	Co. F, 7th NCST
11	Stallings, Oliver C. (5)	Franklin	Co. B, 66th NCT
12	Stamper, William H. (4)	Halifax	Co. D, 43rd NCT

	Date	Limb	Location
1	6 June 1867 8 June 1867 20 June 1867	Arm	CW Military 41 Aud. 6.1, p. 51 CW Military 41
2	15 May 1866 29 May 1866 (2)	Leg	Worth 2, letter Jewett Invoices Aud. 6.1, p. 49
3	12 Sept 1867	Leg	CW Military 41
4	1 May 1866 1 June 1866 24 Aug. 1866 21 Sept 1866 (2)	Leg	Worth 2, Co. List Worth 3, form AG 58, p. 93 Jewett Invoices Aud. 6.1, p. 48
5	21 Feb 1866 18 Sept 1866 12 March 1867 (2)	Arm	Worth 1, Co. List Worth 3, form Jewett Invoices Aud. 6.1, p. 49
6	8 March 1866	Arm	Worth 2, Co. List
7	18 May 1867 31 May 1867	Arm	CW Military 41 Aud. 6.1, p. 51
8	no date 28 Nov 1866 no date	Leg	Worth 8, Co. List CW Military 41 Aud. 6.1, p. 49
9	24 April 1867	Arm	Aud. 6.1, p. 51
10	14 Aug 1867 (2)	Hand	CW Military 41 Aud. 6.1, p. 52
11	29 Sept 1866 2 Oct 1866 29 March 1867 11 May 1867 (2)	Hand	CW Military 41 AG 58, p. 146 CW Military 41 Jewett Invoices Aud. 6.1, p. 50
12	5 March 1866 20 June 1866 25 Oct 1866 (2)	Leg	Worth 2, Co. List Worth 3, form Jewett Invoices Aud. 6.1, p. 48

	Claimant	County	Confederate Unit
1	Stancel, B. (6) (also Stansel)	Robeson	Co. D, 18th NCT
2	Stanly, Jesse (2)	Surry	Co. A, 28th NCT
3	Stanton, A. F.	Granville	Co. E, 15th NCT
4	Starke, James T. (2)	Granville	Co. E, 46th NCT
5	Starnes, David (5) (also Starns)	Union	Co. H, 30th NCT
6	Starnes, H. J.	Union	[Co. E, 48th NCT]
7	Starnes, Thomas H. (4)	Union	Co. B, 43rd NCT
8	Staton, William (4)	Mitchell	Co. C, 10th Bn. NC Heavy Arty.
9	Stephens, John A.	Sampson	Co. D, 38th NCT
10	Stephens, Thomas M. (4)	Rockingham	Co. B, 45th NCT
11	Stevenson, W. M., Capt. (2)	Guilford	
12	Stewart, Coleman (3)	Union	Co. C, 10th Arty. (Co. E, 48th NCT in *NCT Roster*)

	Date	Limb	Location
1	21 Feb 1866 16 Aug 1866 13 Sept 1866 2 Oct 1866 (2) 10 Oct 1866	Leg	Worth 1, Co. List Worth 3, form AG 58, p. 123 Jewett Invoices Aud. 6.1, p. 48 Worth 3, Co. List
2	23 Feb 1867 (2)	Arm	CW Military 41 Aud. 6.1, p. 52
3	2 Oct 1867	Arm	Aud. 6.1, p. 52
4	8 July 1867 (2)	Arm	CW Military 41 Aud. 6.1, p. 52
5	22 Oct 1866 9 Nov 1866 7 Feb 1867 (2) 5 Oct 1867	Leg	Worth 3, Co. List CW Military 41 Jewett Invoices Aud. 6.1, p. 48
6	22 Oct 1866	Arm	Worth 3, Co. List
7	22 Oct 1866 23 March 1867 27 March 1867 27 May 1867	Arm	Worth 3, Co. List CW Military 41 Aud. 6.1, p. 50 CW Military 41
8	23 March 1867 25 March 1867 30 March 1867 3 April 1867	Arm	CW Military 41 Aud. 6.1, p. 50 CW Military 41 CW Military 41
9	15 March 1867	Arm	Aud. 6.1, p. 50
10	12 March 1866 1 Nov 1866 22 Dec 1866 (2)	Leg	CW Mil, Co. List Worth 4, form Jewett Invoices Aud. 6.1, p. 49
11	29 Aug 1866 12 Oct 1866	Leg	AG 58, p. 106 AG 58, p. 170
12	22 Oct 1866 21 Feb. 1867 (2)	Arm	Worth 3, Co. List CW Mil, Co. List Aud. 6.1, p. 49

	Claimant	County	Confederate Unit
1	Stewart, John L. (3) (also Steward)	Moore	Co. D, 49th NCT
2	Stewart, S. J. (2)	Mecklenburg	Co. C, 37th NCT
3	Stewart, Z. M. P. (2)	Johnston	Co. F, 4th NCST
4	Stinson, Abraham (2)	Yadkin	Co. I, 28th NCT
5	Stith, L. A. (3)	Wilson	Asst. Surgeon, 2nd NCST
6	Stone, Atlas	Wake	
7	Stone, Silas M. (3)	Franklin	Co. I, 55th NCT
8	Stowe, J. Green (4) (erroneously listed as Stone on invoice)	Gaston	Co. H, 49th NCT
9	Strickland, Haywood (2)	Cumberland	[Co. B, 20th NCT]
10	Strickland, James B.	Wake	Co. A, 14th NCT
11	Strickland, William D. (4)	Wake	Co. H, 31st NCT
12	Strider, John (2)	Randolph	Co. K, 56th NCT
13	Stroup, Andrew J. (2)	Gaston	Co. H, 56th NCT
14	Stroup, C. W. (2)	Gaston	Co. H, 52nd NCT

	Date	Limb	Location
1	24 Aug 1866 1 Sept 1866 (2)	Leg	AG 58, p. 87 Aud. 6.1, p. 48 Jewett Invoices
2	14 June 1867 (2)	Arm	CW Military 41 Aud. 6.1, p. 52
3	7 June 1867 (2)	Arm	CW Military 41 Aud. 6.1, p. 51
4	1 Feb 1867 (2)	Leg	Jewett Invoices Aud. 6.1, p. 49
5	12 July 1867 23 July 1867 29 July 1867	Arm	CW Military 41 Aud. 6.1, p. 52 CW Military 41
6	no date	Leg	CW Mil, Co. List
7	25 Jan 1866 14 July 1866 24 Aug 1866	Leg	Worth 1, letter Worth 3, letter Aud. 6.1, p. 48
8	no date 1 Sept 1866 22 Nov 1866 (2)	Leg	Worth 8, Co. List AG 58, p. 111 Jewett Invoices Aud. 6.1, p. 48
9	27 March 1867 30 March 1867	Arm	CW Military 41 Aud. 6.1, p. 50
10	24 April 1867	Arm	Aud. 6.1, p. 51
11	16 June 1866 (2) 24 June 1866 no date	Leg	Jewett Invoices Aud. 6.1, p. 49 Worth 2, form CW Mil, Co. List
12	30 Nov 1866 (2)	Leg	Jewett Invoices Aud. 6.1, p. 49
13	no date 24 Aug 1867	Arm	Worth 8, Co. List Aud. 6.1, p. 52
14	20 Sept 1866 (2)	Leg	Aud. 6.1, p. 48 Jewett Invoices

	Claimant	County	Confederate Unit
1	Sturgeon, C. S. (5) (also Stergeon)	Mecklenburg	Co. B, 13th NCT
2	Stutts, A. J. (2)	Montgomery	Co. D, 48th NCT
3	Suit, James A. (5) (Invoice and Aud. list M. as middle initial.)	Person	Co. E, 23rd NCT
4	Summerlin, A. J. (2)	Wayne	Co. G, 55th NCT
5	Summersett, Samuel J.	Brunswick	Co. G, 20th NCT
6	Sumner, Asa (3)	Duplin	Co. B, 3rd NCST
7	Surratt, John (3)	Davidson	Co. F, 7th NCST
8	Sutton, Freeland (2)	Alamance	Co. E, 1st NCST
9	Sutton, John (3)	Lenoir	Co. E, 66th NCT
10	Sutton, W. T.	Sampson	Co. C, 38th NCT
11	Sweaney, A. M. (3) (also Swinney)	Buncombe	Co. B, 7th Ga.
12	Sweaney, Thomas (4)	Person	Co. A, 24th NCT

	Date	Limb	Location
1	13 June 1866 18 Oct 1866 26 Oct 1866 (2) 9 Nov 1866	Leg	Worth 3, form AG 58, p. 186 Jewett Invoices Aud. 6.1, p. 48 Worth 4, Co. List
2	22 April 1867 (2)	Leg	Jewett Invoices Aud. 6.1, p. 49
3	6 June 1866 18 Oct 1866 27 Nov 1866 10 Dec 1866 (2)	Leg	Worth 3, form AG 58, p. 184 Worth 4, Co. List Jewett Invoices Aud. 6.1, p. 49
4	30 March 1867 (2)	Arm	Jewett Invoices Aud. 6.1, p. 50
5	11 March 1880	Hands	Aud. 6.1, p. 52
6	19 April 1866 29 Jan 1867 (2)	Leg	CW Mil, Co. List Jewett Invoices Aud. 6.1, p. 49
7	5 June 1866 1 Feb 1867 (2)	Leg	Worth 3, form Jewett Invoices Aud. 6.1, p. 49
8	10 March 1866 3 March 1867	Arm	Worth 2, Co. List Aud. 6.1, p. 50
9	20 March 1866 25 Aug 1866 (2)	Leg	Worth 2, Co. List Jewett Invoices Aud. 6.1, p. 48
10	30 May 1867	Arm	Aud. 6.1, p. 51
11	10 May 1866 16 Feb 1867 (2)	Arm	Worth 2, Co. List Jewett Invoices Aud. 6.1, p. 49
12	6 June 1866 26 Nov 1866 (2) 27 Nov 1866	Leg	Worth 3, form Jewett Invoices Aud. 6.1, p. 49 Worth 4, Co. List

	Claimant	County	Confederate Unit
1	Swicegood, J. H. (4)	Davidson	Co. A, 54th NCT
2	Swink, Peter J. (3)	Rowan	[Co. K], 8th NCST
3	Tallent, Jesse (2)	Burke	Co. F, 55th NCT
4	Taylor, Abram James (2)	Cumberland	Co. I, 51st NCT
5	Taylor, B. F. (2)	Rockingham	Co. G, 14th NCT
6	Taylor, Benjamin	Stokes	Co. D, 52nd NCT
7	Taylor, George H. (2)	Craven	Co. H, 9th NCST (1st NC Cav.)
8	Taylor, J. W.	Mecklenburg	[Co. B, 53rd NCT]
9	Taylor, Jackson (2)	Moore	Co. H, 30th NCT
10	Taylor, Jesse (4)	Wayne	Co. K, 27th NCT
11	Taylor, John D., Lt. Col. (2)	Brunswick	36th NCT
12	Taylor, John E. (4)	Lenoir	Co. E, 66th NCT
13	Taylor, Lewis (4)	Duplin	Co. A, 30th NCT

	Date	Limb	Location
1	14 June 1866 9 March 1867 (2) 13 March 1867	Leg	Worth 3, form Jewett Invoices Aud. 6.1, p. 48 CW Military 41
2	23 April 1866 21 July 1866 (2)	Leg	CW Mil, Co. List Jewett Invoices Aud. 6.1, p. 48
3	29 Aug 1867 (2)	Arm	CW Military 41 Aud. 6.1, p. 55
4	16 April 1867 20 April 1867	Leg	CW Military 41 Aud. 6.1, p. 54
5	12 March 1866 5 Jan 1870	Arm	CW Mil, Co. List Aud. 6.1, p. 55
6	28 Feb 1867	Arm	Aud. 6.1, p. 54
7	22 Sept 1866 28 Sept 1867	Leg	Worth 3, form Aud. 6.1, p. 53
8	9 Nov 1866	Arm	Worth 4, Co. List
9	29 Aug 1867 4 Sept 1867	Arm	Aud. 6.1, p. 55 Worth 7, form
10	1 Aug 1866 16 Jan 1867 18 Feb 1867 (2)	Leg	Worth 3, form CW Military 41 Jewett Invoices Aud. 6.1, p. 53
11	27 March 1867 (2)	Arm	CW Military 41 Aud. 6.1, p. 54
12	20 March 1866 10 July 1866 11 March 1867 (2)	Leg	Worth 2, Co. List CW Military 41 Jewett Invoices Aud. 6.1, p. 53
13	29 April 1867 30 April 1867 4 May 1867 1 June 1867	Leg	CW Military 41 Aud. 6.1, p. 54 CW Military 41 CW Military 41

	Claimant	County	Confederate Unit
1	Taylor, Malicha Corbell (6) (Leg returned, Feb-March invoice)	Currituck	Co. G, 59th NCT (4th NC Cav.) (Co. H in *NCT Roster*)
2	Taylor, William T. (2)	Cumberland	Co. B, 56th NCT
3	Tays, S. L. (5) (listed as L. S Tayse in Aud.)	Iredell	Co. E, 49th NCT
4	Temple, A. H.	Wake	Co. D, 26th NCT
5	Terrell, J. J., Lt. (4)	Wake	Co. I, 1st NCST
6	Terry, W. H. (2) (also Teary)	Chatham	Co. G, 26th NCT
7	Tew, J. J.	Sampson	Co. K, 51st NCT
8	Thagard, Alexander (3)	Cumberland	Co. E, 44th NCT
9	Thayer, W. S. (4)	Wake	Co. H, 11th Va.
10	Thomas, George W. (2)	Orange	Co. A, 24th NCT
11	Thomas, Isaiah (4)	Edgecombe	Co. H, 17th NCT

	Date	Limb	Location
1	3 May 1866 12 June 1866 12 Sept 1866 24 Oct 1866 (2) Feb-March 1867	Leg	Worth 2, letter Worth 3, form CW Military 41 Jewett Invoices Aud. 6.1, p. 53 Jewett Invoices
2	1 Sept 1866 7 Sept 1867	Leg	Worth 3, form Aud. 6.1, p. 53
3	3 April 1866 9 Oct 1866 13 Feb 1867 27 Feb 1867 (2)	Leg	Worth 2, Co. List CW Military 41 CW Military 41 Jewett Invoices Aud. 6.1, p. 53
4	19 May 1867	Arm	Aud. 6.1, p. 54
5	21 May 1866 2 June 1866 (2) no date	Leg	CW Military 41 Jewett Invoices Aud. 6.1, p. 53 CW Mil, Co. List
6	5 Dec 1866 29 Jan 1867	Leg	Worth 4, Co. List Aud. 6.1, p. 53
7	19 March 1867	Arm	Aud. 6.1, p. 54
8	10 June 1867 13 July 1867	Arm	CW Military 41 Aud. 6.1, p. 54
9	23 May 1866 18 June 1866 23 June 1866 (2)	Leg	Worth 2, form CW Military 41 Jewett Invoices Aud. 6.1, p. 53
10	3 Dec 1867 5 Dec 1867	Arm	CW Military 41 Aud. 6.1, p. 55
11	2 April 1867 4 April 1867 7 Sept 1867 5 Oct 1867	Arm	CW Military 41 Aud. 6.1, p. 54 CW Military 41 CW Military 41

	Claimant	County	Confederate Unit
1	Thomas, J. M. B. (3) (Aud. lists V instead of B as final initial.)	Moore	Co. F, 50th NCT
2	Thomas, John	Anson	Co. H, 43rd NCT
3	Thomas, John T.	Guilford	Co. G, 47th NCT
4	Thomason, Logan (3)	Yancey	Co. C, 16th NCT
5	Thompson, A. G. (3)	Rutherford	Co. A, 39th NCT
6	Thompson, Charles M. (4)	Davidson	Co. I, 14th NCT
7	Thompson, H. W.	Wayne	Co. D, 4th NCST
8	Thomson, F. M.	Orange	Co. A, 66th NCT
9	Thornton, Robert B. (4)	Warren	Co. F, 12th NCT
10	Thrower, J. T. (5) (also T. J.) (Name given as Jeff in NCT Roster; his full name may have been Thomas Jefferson.)	Mecklenburg	Co. H, 11th NCT
11	Tickle, Charles Alexander (5) (also Tickert, Ticker, and Tickl)	Alamance	Co. K, 47th NCT
12	Tiddy, James, Lt. (3)	Mecklenburg	Co. E, 34th NCT

	Date	Limb	Location
1	28 July 1866 11 Aug 1866 (2)	Foot	CW Military 41 Jewett Invoices Aud. 6.1, p. 53
2	12 March 1868	Arm	Aud. 6.1, p. 55
3	23 May 1867	Leg	Aud. 6.1, p. 54
4	7 April 1866 15 Jan 1867 8 Feb 1867	Leg	Worth 2, Co. List CW Military 41 Aud. 6.1, p. 55
5	11 Jan 1867 31 May 1867 (2)	Leg	CW Military 41 Jewett Invoices Aud. 6.1, p. 53
6	2 June 1866 23 Feb. 1867 6 April 1867 (2)	Arm	CW Military 41 CW Military 41 Jewett Invoices Aud. 6.1, p. 54
7	22 May 1867	Arm	Aud. 6.1, p. 54
8	24 April 1867	Arm	Aud. 6.1, p. 54
9	11 July 1866 20 July 1866 (2) no date	Leg	CW Military 41 Jewett Invoices Aud. 6.1, p. 53 CW Military 41
10	10 July 1866 23 July 1866 24 Aug 1866 (2) 9 Nov 1866	Leg	Worth 3, form CW Military 41 Jewett Invoices Aud. 6.1, p. 53 Worth 4, Co. List
11	10 March 1866 27 Oct 1866 1 Nov 1866 4 Dec 1866 6 Dec 1866	Leg	Worth 2, Co. List Worth 3, form CW Military 41 Aud. 6.1, p. 53 Jewett Invoices
12	17 May 1866 11 June 1866 (2)	Leg	CW Military 41 Jewett Invoices Aud. 6.1, p. 53

	Claimant	County	Confederate Unit
1	Tilley, Robert C. (3)	Orange	Co. E, 31st NCT
2	Tilly, John C. (2)	Ashe	Co. K, 37th NCT
3	Tingen, John R. (3) (also Tinger)	Person	Co. H, 24th NCT
4	Tippett, D. F.	Davidson	Co. D, 14th NCT
5	Tipton, John (2) *(see Elijah Randolph in CW Military 41)	Yancey	[Co. G, 58th NCT]
6	Todd, John (3)	Wilson	Co. C, 43rd NCT
7	Tolley, William H. (3)	Yancey	Co. A, 19th NCT
8	Tomberlin, Eli (4) (also Aley)	Union	Co. E, 9th NCST (1st NC Cav.)
9	Tomlin, S. H.	Stokes	Co. H, 22nd NCT
10	Torrence, A. P.	Mecklenburg	[Co. C, 37th NCT]
11	Townsend, C. F. (5)	Robeson	Co. E, 51st NCT
12	Townsend, Fuller (2)	Robeson	[Co. E, 51st NCT]
13	Travelstret, Reuben (3) (also Travenstredt)	Catawba	Co. E. 57th NCT
14	Trice, Charles W.	Wake	[Co. A, 7th Texas]

	Date	Limb	Location
1	15 June 1866 22 Aug 1866 (2)	Leg	CW Military 41 Jewett Invoices Aud. 6.1, p. 53
2	9 Feb 1867 (2)	Leg	CW Military 41 Aud. 6.1, p. 53
3	27 Nov 1866 25 March 1867 6 June 1867	Arm	Worth 4, Co. List CW Military 41 Aud. 6.1, p. 54
4	11 March 1867	Arm	Aud. 6.1, p. 54
5	31 Aug 1867 2 Oct 1867	Arm	CW Military 41* Aud. 6.1, p. 55
6	9 Jan 1867 23 Jan 1867 (2)	Leg	CW Military 41 Jewett Invoices Aud. 6.1, p. 53
7	7 April 1866 8 Dec 1866 (2)	Leg	Worth 2, Co. List CW Military 41 Aud. 6.1, p. 53
8	22 Oct 1866 25 Feb 1867 (2) 24 Sept 1867	Arm	Worth 3, Co. List CW Military 41 Aud. 6.1, p. 54 Worth 7, letter
9	14 March 1867	Leg	Aud. 6.1, p. 54
10	9 Nov 1866		Worth 4, Co. List
11	1 Aug 1867 16 Aug 1867 (2) 26 Aug 1867 5 Sept 1867	Arm	CW Military 41 Aud. 6.1, p. 55 CW Military 41 Aud. 6.1, p. 55 CW Military 41
12	21 Feb 1866 10 Oct 1866	Arm	Worth 1, Co. List Worth 3, Co. List
13	24 Feb 1866 15 July 1867 23 July 1867	Arm	Worth 1, Co. List CW Military 41 Aud. 6.1, p. 54
14	26 April 1867	Arm	Worth 5, letter

	Claimant	County	Confederate Unit
1	Trogden, S. W. (2) (also Trogdon)	Randolph	Co. M, 22nd NCT
2	Troutman, N. B. (4)	Rowan	Co. K, 4th NCT
3	True, John H. (2)	Person	Co. G, 15th NCT
4	Trull, Andrew (2)	Union	[Co. A], 48th NCT
5	Trull, James H. (3)	Union	Co. I, 53rd NCT
6	Tucker, George (2)	Stanly	Co. D, 37th NCT
7	Tucker, William T. (2)	Anson	Co. A, 23rd NCT
8	Tunstall, Patrick A. (6)	Granville	Co. G, 23rd NCT
9	Turner, A. N. (4)	Cleveland	Co. K, 18th NCT
10	Turner, E. D.	Stanly	Co. G, 4th NCST
11	Turner, J. McLeod, Lt. Col. (4)	Davidson	7th NCST

	Date	Limb	Location
1	26 Nov 1867 (2)	Leg	Jewett Invoices Aud. 6.1, p. 53
2	23 April 1866 11 June 1866 3 July 1866 (2)	Leg	CW Mil, Co. List CW Military 41 Jewett Invoices Aud. 6.1, p. 53
3	27 Nov 1866 27 Feb 1867	Arms	Worth 4, Co. List Aud. 6.1, p. 54
4	22 Oct 1866 2 March 1867	Arm	Worth 3, Co. List Aud. 6.1, p. 54
5	22 Oct 1866 21 Feb 1867 (2)	Arm	Worth 3, Co. List CW Mil, Co. List Aud. 6.1, p. 54
6	23 May 1867 29 May 1867	Leg	CW Military 41 Aud. 6.1, p. 54
7	27 May 1867 23 Jan 1868	Arm	CW Military 41 Aud. 6.1, p. 55
8	11 Aug 1866 15 Aug 1866 22 Sept 1866 3 Oct 1866 (2) 5 Sept 1867	Leg	Worth 3, form CW Military 41 AG 58, p. 136 Jewett Invoices Aud. 6.1, p. 53 CW Military 41
9	6 May 1867 23 May 1867 4 June 1867 8 June 1867	Leg	Worth 5, letter CW Military 41 Aud. 6.1, p. 54 CW Military 41
10	17 April 1867	Leg and Arm	Aud. 6.1, p. 55
11	2 July 1867 5 July 1867 5 Aug 1867 23 Aug 1867	Leg	Worth 6, letter Worth 6, letter CW Military 41 Aud. 6.1, p. 54

	Claimant	County	Confederate Unit
1	Turner, Pinckney L. (5)	Catawba	Co. A, 23rd NCT
2	Tuttle, Gideon	Stokes	Co. D, 52nd NCT
3	Tuttle, John F. (3)	Camden	Co. B, 32nd NCT
4	Tysinger, Alexander (4)	Davidson	Co. A, 21st NCT
5	Tyson, ——	Bladen	
6	Tyson, Joseph W. (5)	Bladen	Co. H, 51st NCT
7	Tyson, T. B. (3)	Chatham	Co. I, 32nd NCT
8	Underhill, J. J.	Wayne	Co. C, 2nd NCST
9	Underhill, James D. (2)	Wake	Co. H, 31st NCT
10	Utley, Frank	Wake	
11	Utley, William F. (3)	Wake	Co. D, 26th NCT
12	Vandervoort, William	Rowan	Co. H, 23rd NCT
13	Vann, John R. (4)	Duplin	Co. A, 51st NCT

	Date	Limb	Location
1	24 Feb 1866 26 Nov 1866 29 Nov 1866 16 Jan 1867 (2)	Leg	Worth 1, Co. List CW Military 41 CW Military 41 Jewett Invoices Aud. 6.1, p. 53
2	28 Feb 1867	Arm	Aud. 6.1, p. 54
3	30 Oct 1867 5 Nov 1867 30 Nov 1867	Arm	CW Military 41 Aud. 6.1, p. 55 CW Military 41
4	11 June 1866 1 Nov 1866 13 Nov 1866 17 Nov 1866	Leg	Worth 3, form CW Military 41 Jewett Invoices Aud. 6.1, p. 53
5	9 Feb 1867	Leg	CW Mil, Co. List
6	10 April 1866 22 June 1866 28 Dec 1866 13 Feb 1867 (2)	Leg	Worth 2, Co. List Worth 3, form CW Military 41 Jewett Invoices Aud. 6.1, p. 53
7	5 Dec 1866 6 June 1867 7 June 1867	Arm	Worth 4, Co. List CW Military 41 Aud. 6.1, p. 54
8	22 May 1867	Leg	Aud. 6.1, p. 56
9	no date 18 May 1867	Arm	CW Mil, Co. List Aud. 6.1, p. 56
10	no date	Leg	CW Mil, Co. List
11	14 May 1866 31 May 1866 (2)	Leg	CW Military 41 Jewett Invoices Aud. 6.1, p. 56
12	15 April 1867	Arm	Aud. 6.1, p. 56
13	19 April 1866 26 March 1867 21 April 1867 13 May 1867	Arm	CW Mil, Co. List CW Military 41 Aud. 6.1, p. 56 CW Military 41

	Claimant	County	Confederate Unit
1	Vannoy, W. W. (2)	Wilkes	Co. B, 1st NCST
2	Vestal, O. D. (2)	Chatham	Co. E, 26th NCT
3	Vick, E. C. (3)	Nash	Co. E, 7th NCST
4	Vick, Exum R. (3)	Nash	Co. I, 30th NCT
5	Vick, Reddin A. (4) (also A. Vick)	Edgecombe	Co. E, 43rd NCT
6	Vincent, John (2)	Orange and Alamance	[Co. K, 6th NCST]
7	Vines, Henry (5)	Brunswick	[3rd Co. G], 36th NCT
8	Vinson, G. W.	Chatham	Co. G, 26th NCT
9	Waddell, James H.	Wilson	Co. H, 41st Miss.
10	Wade, J. W.	Montgomery	Co. E, 28th NCT
11	Walker, ____	Halifax	
12	Walker, George W. (2)	New Hanover	Co. C, 59th NCT (4th NC Cav.)
13	Walker, H. J. (4)	Mecklenburg	Co. B, 13th NCT
14	Walker, J. W.	Granville	Co. I, 55th NCT
15	Walker, L. J. (4)	Mecklenburg	Co. B, 13th NCT

	Date	Limb	Location
1	17 June 1867 (2)	Eye	CW Military 41
2	11 July 1867 (2)	Arm	CW Military 41 Aud. 6.1, p. 56
3	24 July 1866 10 Aug 1866 (2)	Leg	CW Military 41 Jewett Invoices Aud. 6.1, p. 56
4	23 July 1866 10 Aug 1866 24 Aug 1866	Leg	CW Military 41 Aud. 6.1, p. 56 Jewett Invoices
5	11 Feb 1867 1 April 1867 3 April 1867 27 May 1867	Leg	CW Military 41 CW Military 41 Aud. 6.1, p. 56 CW Military 41
6	27 Feb 1867 2 March 1867	Arm	CW Military 41 Aud. 6.1, p. 56
7	6 June 1866 25 June 1866 (2) 10 Sept 1879	Both legs	Worth 3, orders (2) Jewett Invoices Aud. 6.1, p. 56 Aud. 6.113
8	8 April 1867	Arm	Aud. 6.1, p. 56
9	29 April 1867	Arm	Aud. 6.1, p. 59
10	31 July 1867	Arm	Aud. 6.1, p. 60
11	5 March 1866	Leg	Worth 2, Co. List
12	9 June 1867 22 June 1867	Arm	Aud. 6.1, p. 59 CW Military 41
13	30 May 1866 20 July 1866 (2) 9 Nov 1866	Leg	Worth 2, form Jewett Invoices Aud. 6.1, p. 57 Worth 4, Co. List
14	8 April 1867	Arm	Aud. 6.1, p. 59
15	30 May 1866 23 July 1866 (2) 9 Nov 1866	Leg	Worth 2, form Jewett Invoices Aud. 6.1, p. 57 Worth 4, Co. List

	Claimant	County	Confederate Unit
1	Walker, Noah J. (3)	Wilson	Co. C, 43rd NCT
2	Walker, William T. (2)	Caswell	Co. H, 6th NCST
3	Walkup, H. C. (3)	Union	Co. B, 26th NCT
4	Wall, M. T. (2)	Johnston	Co. C, 1st NCST
5	Wallace, D. S.	Gaston	Co. H, 23rd NCT
6	Walls, Montraville (2)	Davie	Co. C, 4th NCST
7	Walter, D. P. (4)	Cabarrus	Co. C, 33rd NCT
8	Walters, Edward P. (3)	Granville and Person	Co. E, 35th NCT
9	Ward, Joseph T. (4)	Pitt	Co. E, 27th NCT
10	Ward, W. H.	Orange	Co. G, 44th NCT
11	Warlick, F. T.	Cleveland	Co. C, 55th NCT
12	Warlick, Noah B. (3)	Cleveland	Co. F, 55th NCT
13	Warren, John (2)	Wake	Co. E, 14th NCT
14	Warren, Seymour (4)	Nash	Co. A, 47th NCT

	Date	Limb	Location
1	13 Dec 1866 29 Jan 1867 (2)	Leg	CW Military 41 Jewett Invoices Aud. 6.1, p. 57
2	20 Feb 1866 25 May 1867	Arm	Worth 1, Co. List Aud. 6.1, p. 59
3	15 March 1867 27 March 1867 12 April 1867	Arm	CW Military 41 Aud. 6.1, p. 58 CW Military 41
4	2 March 1867 (2)	Leg	CW Military 41 Aud. 6.1, p. 57
5	19 March 1867	Arm	Aud. 6.1, p. 58
6	15 Oct 1867 (2)	Hand	CW Military 41 Aud. 6.1, p. 60
7	1 Sept 1866 5 Sept 1866 12 Oct 1866 (2)	Leg	Worth 3, letter Worth 3, letter Jewett Invoices Aud. 6.1, p. 57
8	27 Nov 1866 8 May 1867 28 May 1867	Arm	Worth 4, Co. List CW Military 41 Aud. 6.1, p. 59
9	10 Aug 1866 1 Sept 1866 25 Sept 1866 (2)	Leg	Worth 3, letter AG 58, p. 112 Jewett Invoices Aud. 6.1, p. 57
10	22 May 1867	Arm	Aud. 6.1, p. 59
11	23 April 1867	Arm	Aud. 6.1, p. 59
12	no date 25 Oct 1866 19 Dec 1866	Leg	Worth 8, Co. List Worth 3, letter Aud. 6.1, p. 57
13	3 June 1867 (2)	Arm	CW Military 41 Aud. 6.1, p. 59
14	23 July 1866 11 Aug 1866 13 Aug 1866 (2)	Leg	CW Military 41 AG 58, p. 71 Jewett Invoices Aud. 6.1, p. 57

	Claimant	County	Confederate Unit
1	Waters, John A., Sgt. (4) *(includes oath of allegiance)	Rutherford	Co. C, 15th NCT
2	Watkins, David (2)	Wake	Co. E, 14th NCT
3	Watkins, James D.	Stanly	[Co. I, 52nd NCT]
4	Watkins, James R. (6)	Warren	Co. G, 43rd NCT
5	Watkins, W. W.	Wake	Co. E, 41st NCT
6	Watson, Matthew. M. (6)	Robeson	Cobb's Artillery
7	Watts, E. C.	Stanly	Co. H, 8th NCST
8	Weathers, John A. (3)	Lincoln	Co. H, 52nd NCT
9	Weeks, William (4)	Rutherford	Co. C, 34th NCT
10	Wells, D. J. (3)	New Hanover	Co. I, 18th NCT
11	Wells, William B. (2)	Duplin	Co. L, 67th NCT
12	Werner, John	Forsyth	

	Date	Limb	Location
1	12 June 1865* 13 May 1867 29 June 1868 (2)	Leg	CW Military 41 CW Military 41 TC $ Bk 4, p. 95 Aud. 6.1, p. 60
2	no date 25 Feb 1867	Arm	CW Mil, Co. List CW Military 41
3	24 Feb 1866	Leg	Worth 1, Co. List
4	4 June 1866 12 June 1866 11 July 1866 8 Aug 1866 20 Aug 1866 (2)	Leg	CW Military 41 AG 58, p. 11 Worth 3, letter AG 58, p. 58 Jewett Invoices Aud. 6.1, p. 57
5	1 May 1867	Arm	Aud. 6.1, p. 59
6	21 Feb 1866 14 Aug 1866 18 Aug 1866 22 Sept 1866 8 Oct 1866 10 Oct 1866	Leg	Worth 1, Co. List Worth 3, form Worth 3, letter AG 58, p. 131 Aud. 6.1, p. 57 Jewett Invoices
7	4 June 1867	Arm	Aud. 6.1, p. 59
8	27 May 1867 1 June 1867 8 June 1867	Arm	CW Military 41 Aud. 6.1, p. 59 CW Military 41
9	15 Jan 1867 (2) 28 March 1867 (2)	Leg	Worth 4, letter CW Military 41 Jewett Invoices Aud. 6.1, p. 57
10	23 Oct 1866 28 Nov 1866 (2)	Leg	Worth 3, letter Jewett Invoices Aud. 6.1, p. 57
11	19 April 1866 26 Feb 1867	Arm	CW Mil, Co. List Aud. 6.1, p. 58
12	8 March 1866	Leg and Arm	Worth 2, Co. List

	Claimant	County	Confederate Unit
1	Wester, A. H. (3) (Listed as Webster on invoice, though he is likely Archibald H. Westray.)	Nash	Co. I, 30th NCT
2	Whaley, James	Lenoir	[Co. K, 61st NCT]
3	Whaley, Phineas (4)	Lenoir and Wayne	Co. K, 61st NCT
4	Wharton, John W. (3) (also Whorton)	Guilford	Co. M, 21st NCT
5	Wheeler, C. C. (2)	Granville	[Co. I], 63rd NCT (5th NC Cav.)
6	Wheeler, H. C.	Forsyth	Co. G, 12th NCT
7	Wheeler, Jesse (3)	Guilford	Co. K, 45th NCT
8	Wheeler, Oliver C. (3)	Guilford	Co. E, 22nd NCT
9	Wheeler, William S. (3)	Guilford	Co. G, 22nd NCT
10	Wheless, John	Anson	Co. I, 43rd NCT
11	Whisnant, E. M. (3)	Cleveland	Co. E, 12th NCT
12	Whisnant, Morgan (2)	Cleveland	
13	Whitaker, G. Charles (2)	Surry	[Co. F], 21st NCT

	Date	Limb	Location
1	23 July 1866 20 Nov 1866 (2)	Leg	Worth 3, letter Jewett Invoices Aud. 6.1, p. 57
2	20 March 1866	Leg	Worth 2, Co. List
3	10 July 1866 6 Oct 1866 15 Nov 1866 (2)	Leg	Worth 3, letter AG 58, p. 158 Jewett Invoices Aud. 6.1, p. 57
4	16 Feb 1867 no date (2)	Leg	Aud. 6.1, p. 58 Worth 8, Co. List and City List
5	7 May 1867 4 June 1867	Leg	CW Military 41 Aud. 6.1, p. 59
6	16 April 1867	Arm	Aud. 6.1, p. 59
7	12 March 1867 no date (2)	Arm	Aud. 6.1, p. 58 Worth 8, Co. List and City List
8	16 March 1867 no date (2)	Arm	Aud. 6.1, p. 60 Worth 8, Co. List and City List
9	12 March 1867 no date (2)	Arm	Aud. 6.1, p. 58 Worth 8, Co. List and City List
10	1 May 1867	Arm	Aud. 6.1, p. 59
11	28 Nov 1866 17 Jan 1867 (2)	Leg	CW Military 41 Jewett Invoices Aud. 6.1, p. 57
12	no date 24 Nov 1866	Leg	Worth 8, Co. List Worth 4, letter
13	23 Feb 1867 (2)	Arm	CW Military 41 Aud. 6.1, p. 60

	Claimant	County	Confederate Unit
1	Whitaker, T. L. (5)	Halifax	Co. D, 24th NCT
2	White, James R. (2)	Hertford	Co. C, 3rd Bn. NC Light Arty.
3	White, Philo P. (3)	Cabarrus	Co. A, 20th NCT
4	White, T. A.	Mecklenburg	Co. A, 4th NCST
5	Whitener, L. M. (2)	Haywood	Co. K, 46th NCT
6	Whitener, Peter W. (5) (also Whitner)	Catawba	Co. A, 12th NCT
7	Whiteside, J. L. (3)	Rutherford	Co. D, 34th NCT
8	Whitfield, John W. (3)	Duplin	Co. C, 27th NCT
9	Whitfield, W. T. (3)	Chatham	Co. D, 15th NCT
10	Whitley, Daniel (5)	Martin	Co. H, 27th NCT
11	Whitley, Michael (4)	Wake	Co. I, 16th Bn. NC Cav.
12	Whitley, Thomas L. (2)	Martin	[Co. K, 10th NCST (1st NC Arty.)]

	Date	Limb	Location
1	19 Dec 1866 27 June 1867 15 Aug 1867 (2) 6 Nov 1867	Arm	CW Military 41 Worth 6, letter Worth 6, letters Aud. 6.1, p. 60
2	26 June 1867 1 July 1867	Leg	CW Military 41 Aud. 6.1, p. 60
3	26 March 1866 7 April 1866 26 May 1866	Leg	Worth 2, Co. List Worth 2, 7 April Aud. 6.1, p. 57
4	3 April 1867	Arm	Aud. 6.1, p. 58
5	3 Aug 1867 11 Sept 1867	Arm	CW Military 41 Aud. 6.1, p. 60
6	24 Feb 1866 28 Nov 1866 29 Nov 1866 8 Jan 1867 (2)	Leg	Worth 1, Co. List CW Military 41 Aud. 6.1, p. 57 Jewett Invoices
7	28 Feb 1867 5 March 1867 (2)	Leg	CW Military 41 Jewett Invoices Aud. 6.1, p. 58
8	19 April 1866 25 March 1867 29 March 1867	Arm	CW Mil, Co. List CW Military 41 Aud. 6.1, p. 58
9	8 March 1867 15 March 1867 18 March 1867	Arm	CW Military 41 Aud. 6.1, p. 58 CW Military 41
10	2 July 1866 10 July 1866 8 Aug 1866 16 Aug 1866 (2)	Leg	Worth 3, form Worth 3, order AG 58, p. 61 Jewett Invoices Aud. 6.1, p. 57
11	no date 8 June 1866 4 March 1867 (2)	Leg	CW Mil, Co. List Worth 3, form CW Military 41 Aud. 6.1, p. 58
12	21 Feb 1867 29 April 1867	Arm	Aud. 6.1, p. 58 CW Military 41

	Claimant	County	Confederate Unit
1	Whitlock, J. H. (2)	Davie	Co. G, 4th NCST
2	Whitlow, William J. (2)	Person	Co. B, 59th NCT (4th NC Cav.)
3	Wicker, B. F.	Moore	Co. D, 61st NCT
4	Wiggs, John H. (4)	Wayne	Co. I, 10th NCST (1st NC Arty.)
5	Wilfong, Sidney T. (4)	Catawba	Co. A, 12th NCT
6	Wilkerson, D. M.	Orange	Co. E, 36th NCT
7	Wilkerson, D. N.	Orange	Co. E, 31st NCT
8	Wilkinson, Malcom (7) (erroneously listed as Wilkerson in Aud.)	Robeson	Co. E, 51st NCT
9	Williams, Gaston	Forsyth	
10	Williams, J. G.	Forsyth	
11	Williams, John A.	Chatham	Co. H, 6th NCST
12	Williams, John H. (2)	Buncombe	Co. I, 25th NCT
13	Williams, John P.		
14	Williams, Mac.	Yancey	58th NCT
15	Williams, N. L. (5)	Polk	Co. G, 60th NCT

	Date	Limb	Location
1	13 March 1866 12 June 1867	Arm	Worth 2, Co. List Aud. 6.1, p. 60
2	27 Nov 1866 12 March 1867	Arm	Worth 4, Co. List Aud. 6.1, p. 58
3	1 April 1867	Arm	Aud. 6.1, p. 58
4	1 Aug 1866 16 Jan 1867 23 Feb 1867 (2)	Leg	Worth 3, form CW Military 41 Jewett Invoices Aud. 6.1, p. 58
5	24 Feb 1866 25 March 1867 2 April 1867 8 April 1867	Arm	Worth 1, Co. List CW Military 41 Aud. 6.1, p. 58 CW Military 41
6	1 May 1867	Arm	Aud. 6.1, p. 59
7	20 April 1867	Arm	Aud. 6.1, p. 59
8	21 Feb 1866 4 July 1866 18 Aug 1866 22 Sept 1866 10 Oct 1866 18 Oct 1866 (2)	Leg	Worth 1, Co. List Worth 3, form Worth 3, letter AG 58, p. 138 Worth 3, Co. List Jewett Invoices Aud. 6.1, p. 57
9	8 March 1866	Leg	Worth 2, Co. List
10	20 May 1867		CW Military 41
11	12 June 1867	Arm	Aud. 6.1, p. 60
12	10 May 1866 30 May 1867	Arm	Worth 2, Co. List Aud. 6.1, p. 59
13	13 Feb. 1869	Arm	TC $ Bk 4, p. 199
14	2 March 1867	Eyes	Aud. 6.1, p. 58
15	17 April 1866 31 Jan 1867 20 Feb 1867 26 Feb 1867 (2)	Leg	Worth 2, Co. List CW Military 41 CW Military 41 Jewett Invoices Aud. 6.1, p. 58

	Claimant	County	Confederate Unit
1	Williams, S. G.	Rowan	
2	Williams, Thomas A.	Orange	Co. G, 44th NCT
3	Williams, Tyre (2)	Forsyth	Co. K, 33rd NCT
4	Williamson, Samuel A. (2)	Sampson	Co. C, 1st NCST
5	Williamson, Thomas A.	Orange	Co. G, 44th NCT
6	Willis, Henry C. (3)	Guilford	Co. B, 45th NCT
7	Wilson, J. H.	Davidson	Co. I, 14th NCT
8	Wilson, R. E. (5) (listed both as a major and a captain)	Rowan and Yadkin	[Co. A], 1st Bn. NC Sharpshooters
9	Wilson, Samuel (2) (also Willson)	Yancey	[Co. C], 16th NCT
10	Wimmer, John (5)	Forsyth	Co. K, 48th NCT
11	Winberry, William J. (2) (also Windberry)	Martin	Co. B, 44th NCT
12	Winfree, John H. (3)	Halifax	Co. D, 43rd NCT
13	Winstead, Theophilus T. (3) (also Winsted)	Nash	Co. I, 30th NCT
14	Wise, Franklin (2)	Catawba	Co. G, 57th NCT
15	Withers, Auston	Mecklenburg	
16	Withers, Benjamin A.	Mecklenburg	Co. A, 11th NCT

	Date	Limb	Location
1	23 April 1866	Leg	CW Mil, Co. List
2	5 April 1867	Arm	Aud. 6.1, p. 58
3	8 May 1867 11 May 1867	Leg	CW Military 41 Aud. 6.1, p. 59
4	21 June 1867 (2)	Arm	CW Military 41 Aud. 6.1, p. 60
5	20 April 1867	Arm	Aud. 6.1, p. 59
6	no date 5 Sept 1866 6 Sept 1867	Leg	Worth 8, Co. List Worth 3, letter Aud. 6.1, p. 57
7	14 March 1867	Arm	Aud. 6.1, p. 58
8	5 Aug 1866 8 Sept 1866 25 Sept 1866 (2) 22 June 1867	Leg	Worth 3, letter AG 58, p. 116 Jewett Invoices Aud. 6.1, p. 57 CW Military 41
9	7 April 1866 27 Feb 1867	Arm	Worth 2, Co. List Aud. 6.1, p. 58
10	25 June 1866 26 June 1866 11 Aug 1866 (2) 4 May 1867	Leg and Arm	Worth 3, form CW Military 41 Jewett Invoices Aud. 6.1, p. 57
11	4 July 1866 22 July 1867	Leg	Worth 3, form Aud. 6.1, p. 57
12	19 July 1867 23 July 1867 25 July 1867	Arm	CW Military 41 Aud. 6.1, p. 60 CW Military 41
13	23 July 1866 12 Jan 1867 (2)	Leg	Worth 3, form Jewett Invoices Aud. 6.1, p. 57
14	25 April 1867 1 May 1867	Arm	Aud. 6.1, p. 59 CW Mil, Co. List
15	9 Nov 1866	Arm	Worth 4, Co. List
16	4 April 1867	Arm	Aud. 6.1, p. 58

	Claimant	County	Confederate Unit
1	Womack, W.	Cleveland	Co. C, 55th NCT
2	Womble, John	Wake	Co. D, 31st NCT
3	Womick, A. B. (2)	Rutherford	Co. G, 5th SC
4	Woodall, George W. (2)	Wake	Co. F, 9th Ark.
5	Woodall, W. W.	Wake	Co. G, 3rd NCST
6	Workman, W. J.	Orange	Co. G, 44th NCT
7	Worley, William (2)	Johnston	Co. C, 24th NCT
8	Wright, G. H.	Cleveland	Co. E, 12th NCT
9	Wright, George	Cleveland	[Co. F, 34th NCT]
10	Wright, N.	Cleveland	Co. F, 34th NCT
11	Wright, Thomas B. (5) *(see also Walter R. Bell in CW Mil. 41)	Duplin	Co. E, 20th NCT
12	Yates, Bradley (2)	Columbus	Co. K, 20th NCT
13	Yates, Lewis	Wake	Co. H, 47th NCT
14	Yount, Reuben L. (3)	Catawba	[Co. E, 32nd NCT]
15	Yount, Sidney L. (2)	Catawba	Co. A, 12th NCT
16	Zimmerman, David (2)	Burke	Co. K, 35th NCT

	Date	Limb	Location
1	8 April 1867	Arm	Aud. 6.1, p. 59
2	11 March 1867	Arm	Aud. 6.1, p. 58
3	2 Oct 1867 (2)	Hand	CW Military 41 Aud. 6.1, p. 60
4	21 May 1867 (2)	Leg	CW Military 41 Aud. 6.1, p. 59
5	21 May 1867	Arm	Aud. 6.1, p. 59
6	2 April 1867	Arm	Aud. 6.1, p. 58
7	5 March 1866 20 Feb 1867	Arm	Worth 2, Co. List Aud. 6.1, p. 57
8	8 April 1867	Arm	Aud. 6.1, p. 59
9	9 March 1868	Hand	CW Military 41
10	4 May 1867	Arm	Aud. 6.1, p. 59
11	19 April 1866 25 March 1867 2 April 1867 6 April 1867 6 June 1867	Arm	CW Mil, Co. List CW Military 41* Aud. 6.1, p. 58 CW Military 41 CW Military 41
12	21 Feb 1867 26 Feb 1867	Arm	CW Military 41 Aud. 6.1, p. 61
13	23 April 1867	Arm	Aud. 6.1, p. 61
14	24 Feb 1866 22 Feb 1867 2 March 1867	Arm	Worth 1, Co. List CW Military 41 Aud. 6.1, p. 61
15	24 Feb 1866 23 April 1867	Arm	Worth 1, Co. List Aud. 6.1, p. 61
16	25 June 1867 (2)	Hand	CW Military 41 Aud. 6.1, p. 61

Bibliography

Adjutant Generals Records. State Archives, Office of Archives and History, Raleigh.

Arkansas, State of. *Acts of the General Assembly of the State of Arkansas.* Little Rock: Woodruff and Blocher, 1867.

"Artificial Limbs and How to Make Them." *Confederate States Medical and Surgical Journal* 1 (April 1864).

"Association to Purchase Artificial Limbs for Maimed Soldiers." *Confederate States Medical and Surgical Journal* 1 (April 1864).

Barja, Roberto H., and Richard A. Sherman. *What to Expect When You Lose a Limb.* Washington, D.C.: U.S. Government Printing Office, 1986.

Camp, David M. *The American Yearbook and National Register for 1869.* Hartford: O. D. Case and Company, 1869.

Chisolm, J. Julian. *A Manual of Military Surgery.* 3d ed. 1864. Reprint, Dayton: Morningside Press, 1992.

Clark, Walter, ed. *Histories of the Several Regiments and Battalions from North Carolina in the Great War, 1861-'65.* 5 vols. Raleigh and Goldsboro: State of North Carolina, 1901.

Correspondence Relating to Artificial Limbs, 1866-1869. Civil War Collection, Military Collection. State Archives, Office of Archives and History, Raleigh.

Cumming, Kate. *Kate: The Journal of a Confederate Nurse.* Edited by Richard Barksdale Harwell. Baton Rouge: Louisiana State University Press, 1959.

Cunningham, H. H. *Doctors in Gray.* 1958. Reprint, Baton Rouge: Louisiana State University Press, 1993.

Daily Standard (Raleigh).

Duffy, John. *The Healers: A History of American Medicine.* Urbana: University of Illinois Press, 1987.

Figg, Laurann. "Clothing Adaptations of Civil War Amputees." Master's thesis, Iowa State University, 1990.

Figg, Laurann, and Jane Farrell-Beck. "Amputation in the Civil War: Physical and Social Dimensions." Unpublished manuscript, Vesterheim Museum, Decorah, Iowa, 1993.

Fisher, Clyde Olin. "A Brief History of Confederate Pensions and Soldiers' Relief in North Carolina." Master's thesis, Columbia University, 1916.

Fishman, Sidney. "Amputation." In *Psychological Practices with the Physically Disabled*, edited by James F. Garnett and Edna S. Levine. New York: Columbia University Press, 1962.

Foster, Gaines M. *Ghosts of the Confederacy*. New York: Oxford University Press, 1987.

Friedman, Lawrence W. *The Psychological Rehabilitation of the Amputee*. Springfield, Ill.: Charles C. Thomas, 1978.

General Assembly Session Records. State Archives, Office of Archives and History, Raleigh.

Georgia, State of. *Acts and Resolutions of the General Assembly of the State of Georgia, 1878-1879*. Atlanta: James P. Harrison, 1880.

Kuz, Julian E., and Bradley P. Bengston. *Orthopaedic Injuries of the Civil War*. Kennesaw, Ga.: Kennesaw Mountain Press, 1996.

Letter Book of the Superintendent of the Department of Artificial Limbs. Adjutant Generals Records. State Archives, Office of Archives and History, Raleigh.

Linderman, Gerald F. *Embattled Courage: The Experience of Combat in the Civil War*. New York: Free Press, 1987.

Manarin, Louis H., and Weymouth T. Jordan Jr., comps. *North Carolina Troops: A Roster*. 15 vols. to date. Raleigh: Division of Archives and History, Department of Cultural Resources, 1966-.

Maughs, G. M. B. "Thoughts on Surgery, Operative and Conservative, suggested by a visit to the Battle-field and Hospitals of the Army of Tennessee." *Confederate States Medical and Surgical Journal* 1 (September 1864).

McCawley, Patrick J. *Artificial Limbs for Confederate Soldiers*. Columbia: South Carolina Department of Archives and History, 1992.

McDaid, Jennifer Davis. "With Lame Legs and No Money." *Virginia Cavalcade* (winter 1998).

Minor, James M. "Report on Artificial Limbs." *Bulletin of the New York Academy of Medicine* 1 (1861).

Mississippi, State of. *Journal of the House of Representatives of the State of Mississippi*. Jackson: J. J. Shannon and Company, 1866.

North Carolina, State of. *Journal of the Senate of the General Assembly of the State of North Carolina at its Session of 1866-'67*. Raleigh: William E. Pell, 1867.

Raleigh Sentinel.

Shaffner Diary and Papers. Private Collections. State Archives, Office of Archives and History, Raleigh.

Texas, State of. *Journal of the House of Representatives of the Eleventh Legislature*. Austin: State Gazette, 1866.

Treasurer's Cash Book 4, 1865-1871. Treasurer's and Comptroller's Papers. State Archives, Office of Archives and History, Raleigh.

Wiley, Bell I. *The Life of Johnny Reb*. Baton Rouge: Louisiana State University, 1994.

Worth, Jonathan. Governors Letter Books. State Archives, Office of Archives and History, Raleigh.

——. Governors Papers. State Archives, Office of Archives and History, Raleigh.

——. Papers. Private Collections. State Archives, Office of Archives and History, Raleigh.

Index